To my dear friends, Candy & Raymond Solomon, who kept my spirits high during the writing of this book

Acknowledgments

In our quest to give accurate up-to-date information on conquering impotentence and the breakthrough medications, we have received generous research assistance from a very gifted group of family, friends, and colleagues. We express our gratitude to the following:
Allyn Gauthier, Ashley E. Bruce, Brittnye Bruce, Claire Bruce, Hugh Cruse, MPH, Kimberly McIlwain, MD, Matthew Silliman, Michael McIlwain, Robert G. Bruce, III.

Contents

The *Unofficial Guide* Reader's Bill of Rights

We Give You More Than the Official Line

Welcome to the *Unofficial Guide* series of Lifestyles titles—books that deliver critical, unbiased information that other books can't or won't reveal—*the inside scoop*. Our goal is to provide you with the *most accessible, useful* information and advice possible. The recommendations we offer in these pages are not influenced by the corporate line of any organization or industry; we give you the hard facts, whether those institutions like them or not. If something is ill-advised or will cause a loss of time and/or money, we'll give you ample warning. And if it is a worthwhile option, we'll let you know that, too.

Armed and Ready

Our hand-picked authors confidently and critically report on a wide range of topics that matter to smart readers like you. Our authors are passionate about their subjects, but have distanced themselves enough from them to help you be armed and protected, and help you make educated decisions as you go through your process. It is our intent that, from having read this book, you will avoid the pitfalls everyone else falls into and get it right the first time.

Don't be fooled by cheap imitations; this is the *genuine article Unofficial Guide* series from Macmillan Publishing. You may be familiar with our proven track record of the travel *Unofficial Guides,* which have more than three million copies in print. Each year, thousands of travelers—new and old—are armed with a brand new, fully updated edition of the flagship *Unofficial Guide to Walt Disney World,* by Bob Sehlinger. It is our intention here to provide you with the same level of objective authority that Mr. Sehlinger does in his brainchild.

The Unofficial Panel of Experts

Every work in the Lifestyle *Unofficial Guides* is intensively inspected by a team of top professionals in their fields. These experts review the manuscript for factual accuracy, comprehensiveness, and an insider's determination as to whether the manuscript fulfills the credo in this Reader's Bill of Rights. In other words, our Panel ensures that you are, in fact, getting "the inside scoop."

Our Pledge

The authors, the editorial staff, and the Unofficial Panel of Experts assembled for *Unofficial Guides* are determined to lay out the most valuable alternatives available for our readers. This dictum means that our writers must be explicit, prescriptive, and above all, direct. We strive to be thorough and complete, but our goal is not necessarily to have the "most" or "all" of the information on a topic; this is not, after all, an encyclopedia. Our objective is to help you narrow down your options to the best of what is available, unbiased by affiliation with any industry or organization.

In each *Unofficial Guide* we give you:

- Comprehensive coverage of necessary and vital information
- Authoritative, rigidly fact-checked data
- The most up-to-date insights into trends
- Savvy, sophisticated writing that's also readable
- Sensible, applicable facts and secrets that only an insider knows

Special Features

Every book in our series offers the following six special sidebars in the margins that are devised to help you get things done cheaply, efficiently, and smartly.

1. "Timesaver"—tips and shortcuts that save you time.
2. "Moneysaver"—tips and shortcuts that save you money.
3. "Watch Out!"—more serious cautions and warnings.
4. "Bright Idea"—general tips and shortcuts to help you find an easier or smarter way to do something.
5. "Quote"—statements from real people that are intended to be prescriptive and valuable to you.
6. "Unofficially..."—an insider's fact or anecdote.

We also recognize your need to have quick information at your fingertips, and have thus provided the following comprehensive sections at the back of the book:

1. **Glossary:** Definitions of complicated terminology and jargon.

2. **Resource Guide:** Lists of relevant agenices, associations, institutions, Web sites, etc.
3. **Recommended Reading List:** Suggested titles that can help you get more in-depth information on related topics.
4. **Important Documents:** "Official" pieces of information you need to refer to, such as government forms.
5. **Important Statistics:** Facts and numbers presented at-a-glance for easy reference.
6. **Index.**

Letters, Comments, and Questions from Readers

We strive to continually improve the *Unofficial* series, and input from our readers is a valuable way for us to do that.

Many of those who have used the *Unofficial Guide* travel books write to the authors to ask questions, make comments, or share their own discoveries and lessons. For Lifestyle *Unofficial Guides*, we would also appreciate all such correspondence, both positive and critical, and we will make best efforts to incorporate readers' feedback and comments in revised editions of this work.

How to write to us:

Unofficial Guides
Macmillan Lifestyle Guides
Macmillan Publishing
1633 Broadway
New York, NY 10019
Attention: Readers' Comments

The *Unofficial Guide* Panel of Experts

The *Unofficial Guide* editorial team recognizes that you've purchased this book with the expectation of getting the most authoritative, carefully inspected information currently available. Toward that end, on each and every title in this series, we have selected a minimum of two "official" experts comprising the "Unofficial Panel" who painstakingly review the manuscripts to ensure: factual accuracy of all data; inclusion of the most up-to-date and relevant information; and that, from an insider's perspective, the authors have armed you with all the necessary facts you need—but the institutions don't want you to know.

For *The Unofficial Guide to Conquering Impotence,* we are proud to introduce the following panel of experts:

Laura McIlwain has been training for her medical degree at the University of South Florida College of Medicine with a focus in Internal Medicine. Her research interests include osteoporosis and arthritis. She currently conducts an Osteoarthritis support group for the Arthritis Foundation.

Hugh Cruise is an epidemiologist from the University of South Florida College of Public Health. He currently holds a position as a biological scientist at the H. Lee Moffitt Cancer Center and Research Institute. His research interests include multiple myeloma, osteoporosis, and quality of life issues. His focus in this research is to design, implement, and maintain data systems for research studies.

Introduction: No Longer a Secret

Ever since Viagra, the internationally touted "impotence cure," was approved by the Food and Drug Administration (FDA) in March 1998, telephones in doctors' offices have been ringing nonstop. With Viagra's dramatic release onto the market, the centuries-old taboo of talking about impotency, or erectile dysfunction, was finally shattered.

As with once-censored topics such as sex, birth control, pregnancy, menopause, and even depression, both men and women of all ages can now openly discuss this common urological problem. Nonetheless, with any newly touted "cure" comes a host of amazing promises, as well as a few problems—some serious, some not-so-serious.

The ability to make love plays a vital role in men's lives. And although we assume that sexual intercourse is a natural bodily function for men, the fear of being unable to have or to sustain an erection forces thousands—possibly millions—of men to avoid all sexual contact. As one 59-year-old man said, "I'd rather my wife think I was in a bad mood at night than have her know I could not function as a man."

Many men equate manhood with the ability to perform sexually at will. Hence erectile dysfunction causes them to feel they have lost their masculinity. They neglect their partners, and stay preoccupied with other activities or friends to avoid intimate situations. Sadly, some even choose to divorce or break up long-term dating relationships to keep anyone from knowing the truth.

Having erectile dysfunction or impotence is NO reason to avoid your wife or partner! It's a common problem that almost all men face at some time. It is easy to diagnose and easy to treat.

Relax: You Are Not Alone

If you or someone you love suffers from impotence, it will be comforting to know that you are in great company. Some type of erectile dysfunction affects more than 50 percent of men worldwide aged 40 to 70. This breaks down to one out of every 10 males in the United States, yet only about five percent of the men affected get treatment for their problem. As the baby boomers enter their middle and senior years, these numbers can only increase. The problem is that of these sufferers, an estimated 90 percent don't seek medical help.

What Is Impotence, Anyway?

Impotence is the inability to achieve and maintain an erection that is firm enough or that lasts long enough to have successful sexual intercourse. It is a frustrating condition that may have psychological, medical or physical causes. According to a 1992 National Institutes of Health study of the problem, impotence includes anything from "inability to get an erection" to "unsatisfactory sex performance." There are, however, many types of sexual dysfunction that may be confused with impotence. Impotence does not mean premature ejaculation, low sex drive, or infertility. It is not caused by masturbation or too much sex earlier in life. Also, while most men experience impotence at some time in their lives, it is not normal and can be easily treated.

Before Viagra came on the market, most men never spoke of this problem—not to their doctors, their wives, or to their friends. Impotency was definitely not something discussed in the locker room! The problem is so common that it happens to men younger than 40, yet can be a complaint among men in their eighties. In fact, researchers show that up to 39 percent of men have had some problem with erection by the time they reach 40. This number dramatically increases to about two-thirds of all men by age 70.

A Little Knowledge Goes a Long Way

If you or someone you know is affected by erection problems, there are simple steps you can take to return to a satisfying sex life. Perhaps the first and most important step is admitting to having a problem, then tracking down its cause. Did you know that in most cases, erectile dysfunction is linked to some physical or medical problem? Psychological problems or even old age can cause impotence, but with much less frequency.

Your doctor can determine if there are any underlying problems contributing to difficulty with erection and can help you find the best treatment to restore sexual function. As we explain in Chapter 1, there are ways to find a doctor who is both understanding and empathetic, and with whom you can discuss such intimate and personal concerns without embarrassment.

Understanding Performance Anxiety

Although erection problems are extremely common, men who experience them feel high anxiety and distress. Men tell of questioning their manhood. They worry that the problem will threaten their marriage or other intimate relationships, and many men assume that erectile dysfunction is a sure sign of old age or disease.

These feelings of fear, anxiety, and stress are triggered each time the man fails to perform sexually or even when he thinks about the problem. With each unsuccessful performance, these feelings become a never-ending cycle of fear of failure, stress, depression, and more erection problems. Some of the most common feelings these men have include feeling ill at ease, discontent, anxious, angry, resentful, fearful, inadequate, and frustrated. Other possible problems low self-esteem and insomnia.

When you combine the highly charged fears created by erectile dysfunction with the silence that has for years shrouded male sexual problems, it's no wonder men have had difficulty finding the answers they need to break this vicious cycle that so often results in sexual failure. After failing repeatedly to have an erection, some men simply give up, assume nothing can help, and withdraw from attempting sexual activity. It is not unusual for some men in their sixties or seventies to say they have not had sex in a decade or even two.

You have to remember that your mind is very powerful. Even a normal, healthy man with no physical problems can sabotage his erections simply by worrying about his ability to perform. Some men view impotence as a threat to their manhood, and an enemy of their self-esteem, or as one man put it, "I'm no longer a real man because I cannot perform like I used to in the bedroom."

Along with this self-imposed punishment, men often lean on myths to explain their impotence. Everything from infidelity to masturbation has been blamed for sexual dysfunction, but there is no truth to either of these myths! If you suffer from impotence, you need not suffer any longer, since successful treatment is readily available.

In a random Internet survey regarding men and their feelings about sexual performance, the following statements were given most frequently:

1. Men should never express their true feelings to a woman regarding fears or performance problems.
2. The sexual act is a male's time to perform.
3. A real man is always ready to have sex—any time of day.
4. Only men should initiate sex.
5. Sex means one thing: intercourse.
6. If you cannot have an erection, then you cannot have sex.
7. After you have an orgasm, then the sexual experience has ended.
8. If you ejaculate prematurely, then you are losing your ability to have sex.

Communication Leads to Effective Treatment

Think about it. How is your doctor going to treat a problem you are unwilling to discuss? Also, considering men's traditional reluctance to address erection problems, your doctor may not ask you about it. The problem with this cycle of silence is that millions of men and women are missing a tremendous source of pleasure in their relationships simply because no one wants to ask for help.

Playing Detective: Medications and Alcohol Can Cause Impotence

To find the causes of impotence, you have to be a sleuth. Medications are the first possible suspects as they cause the problem in about 25 percent of all cases. They can affect sexual function and cause erection problems, yet in these cases, impotence is easily conquered simply by stopping the medication. For example, blood pressure medications commonly cause erectile dysfunction, such as beta-blockers and diuretics.

Antidepressants, tranquilizers, anti-anxiety drugs, and lithium can also cause erection problems. As with hypertension medications, you need to alert your doctor before trying another medication.

Too Much Alcohol Relaxes Everything

One of the main causes of impotence may be in that icy mug of beer you are enjoying right now. A common cause of difficulty with erection is overuse of alcohol. Small amounts of alcohol can help us relax and remove inhibitions, which can help the sexual mood and actually increase sexual activity.

Nevertheless, as the amount of alcohol in the blood increases, the alcohol only serves to impair the brain's ability to sense sexual stimulation, leading to loss of the ability to have erections. With longer and steady use of alcohol, there can be damage to nerves that control erection. Excessive use of alcohol can also lead to liver disease and other chronic ailments that make sexual activity and erection more difficult.

One or two drinks daily may be safe for most people. However, everyone is different, so knowing your body is important. This includes knowing when to stop drinking before sexual activity. Some experts recommend using alcohol after sex rather than before if you happen to be sensitive to its effect.

Hypertension Medications Are Also Prime Suspects

An estimated 50 million adult Americans have hypertension, which has no early symptoms. The condition is a major cause of heart disease and stroke—the first and third leading causes of death in this country—and it also can lead to kidney failure. Millions take medication to control hypertension, but did you know that almost every blood pressure medication has been linked at some time with impotence?

The good news is that some high-blood-pressure medications are more problematic than others, so if you think your prescription might be causing an erection problem, talk with your doctor. Perhaps trying another medication is in order. Your doctor may choose from one category of blood pressure medications that is less likely to cause erectile dysfunction. It may even be necessary to try several medications to find the best combination with the fewest side effects. You won't know if this will help your situation unless you ask, so don't let shyness keep you from experiencing total wellness. There are almost always other medications that can control blood pressure that do not cause erectile dysfunction.

Some Drugs Relax More Than You Desired

If performance anxiety is what is causing your impotence, and if tranquilizers help your anxiety, they may promote sexual function and activity simply by removing completely the cause of your problem. However, tranquilizers, sedatives and anti-anxiety drugs can relax you and cause drowsiness. The problem is that they may relax more than you had hoped for!

Furthermore, some tranquilizers may be more likely than others to result in erection problems. Keep in mind that each person is different. You may not discover what works for you until you and your doctor consider a trial of more than one type of medication. If you need tranquilizers, just try to be patient and let your doctor help you find the correct one as quickly as possible.

Antidepressants Can Interrupt Performance

Antidepressants can also cause difficulty with erections. While depression can definitely create erectile dysfunction, it is important to be sure that the medication is not itself leading to impotence. As with tranquilizers, any antidepressant can potentially be the cause of erectile dysfunction. You may need to test more than one to find the best relief with the fewest side effects. Your doctor can guide you to those that are least likely to cause erection problems while offering the most benefit to control depression.

That Antacid May Calm More Than Your Stomach

While medications that alleviate gastric acid, heartburn, and peptic ulcers calm the storm of stomach distress, they leave another undesirable problem in their wake—again, impotence.

Even though these drugs are effective at relieving excess acid, they affect erection by lowering the effectiveness of the male hormone testosterone. Lower levels of testosterone can negatively affect your libido, or sexual drive. These drugs are very commonly used, but many men do not think to tell their doctor they take them.

The good news is that if you have erection problems and are taking a common stomach medication, Viagra may provide an easy solution to this problem.

When Uppers Are Downers

Marijuana, cocaine, heroin, methadone, amphetamines, and other non-prescription drugs can also limit many functions of the body, including sexual function and erections. Cigarette smoking is still another possible culprit when it comes to erectile dysfunction. Not only does smoking increase the chances of atherosclerosis in the arteries that lead to the legs and penis, it decreases the blood flow necessary for an erection to occur. Now there's a reason to finally stop smoking!

The Plot Thickens: Clues to Physical Causes

While most men occasionally experience problems with achieving or maintaining an erection, especially when they are under unusual stress, it is not considered abnormal until it occurs repeatedly. In most of these cases, the specific cause may be entirely correctable. While it was once the general consensus that "impotency is all in your head," we now know that the majority of cases of impotency (80 percent) are caused by some identifiable physical problem.

The Problem of Aging

The most frequent factors resulting in erection difficulty are physical changes associated with aging. Women seem to be in touch with the changes that occur to the female body through the years, but men are often either less aware or simply less concerned. Just as the woman's body undergoes periodic changes, so does the man's. For example, between the ages of 40 and 70, a man loses 12 to 20 pounds of muscle, 15 percent of bone mass, and two inches in height. His body metabolism also slows and, after the age of 40, his testicles shrink slightly and sperm production declines. These changes are accompanied by a thickening of connective tissue that forms in the prostate gland, leading to problems with urination and ejaculation. The functioning of the penis becomes sluggish as the chambers responsible for erection fill with connective tissue and as its supporting arteries narrow.

For some five million men, testosterone levels begin dropping around age 40, resulting in a corresponding decline in traits society equates with manhood. This may be a cause of loss of sexual drive or libido. And while the testosterone loss is subtle compared to the estrogen decline in women, the levels do drop about one percent per year after age 40, resulting in a 30-percent decline by age 70. Believe it or not, some men do experience drops in their testosterone levels severe enough to result in hot flashes and night sweats.

Everyone ages. You can't run from it nor can you stop it. But, there are some things you can do to make the transitions smoother. We will show you how throughout this book.

Diseases Contribute to Dysfunction

Certain medical problems, such as diabetes mellitus, can lead to a higher risk of erection dysfunction and impotence. Diabetes occurs when the body either stops producing insulin or produces less than required, resulting in high blood sugar.

Diabetes can creep up on you, as it has to an estimated 100 million people worldwide. It affects more than 12 million Americans; about four percent of all women and two percent of men in the United States become diabetic. And because the initial symptoms (fatigue, frequent urination, extreme thirst) are usually mild, half of these 12 million Americans do not realize they have diabetes.

About half of all diabetic men have problems with erection, which can be caused by damage to the nerves or from atherosclerosis. This is more common in diabetics.

Another common cause of impotence in men is atherosclerosis, which is hardening of the arteries. This is the process that causes blockages in the coronary arteries that supply the heart muscle itself and can result in heart attack. Atherosclerosis can also affect the arteries leading to or in the brain and can cause stroke.

When atherosclerosis affects the arteries of the legs, it can cause blockage of the blood flow, pain in the calves of the legs when walking, and can also affect the arteries that supply the penis and are critical for developing an erection. Many Americans are afflicted with atherosclerosis, and a high percentage of these are men, making this a leading cause of erectile dysfunction.

The Role of Hormones

Although more important for libido or desire, the male hormone testosterone can also affect erection, resulting in impotence. Testosterone levels in all men commonly lessen with age. However, taking steroids for certain illnesses like chronic obstructive pulmonary disease can also cause testosterone levels to drop. Once testosterone is low, then libido can be diminished.

Other health problems that may also develop with low testosterone levels include osteoporosis, general weakness, and lack of a sense of well-being. These problems can be effectively treated with testosterone supplementation, which can give great relief. That's why it is important to bring problems such as impotence to your doctor's attention. Proper treatment of another serious health problem caused by low testosterone levels may also help you maintain an erection again.

Some hormone deficiencies and abnormalities can also contribute to erection problems and impotence. These include abnormally low thyroid hormone (hypothyroidism), as well as overactive thyroid (hyperthyroidism). Other uncommon problems, such as certain brain tumors, can also be causes of erectile dysfunction. Your doctor can determine if you need to test for these less common causes of erection problems.

Prostate Problems and Nerve-related Diseases

Damage to nerves that supply the prostate and other pelvic organs can also cause impotence. A stroke can damage parts of the brain that send messages via these nerves to the penis. Prostate surgery, especially removal of the prostate for cancer (radical total prostatectomy) damages the nerves that control erection in the majority of patients, although newer surgical techniques can lower the risk of nerve damage to about 50 percent.

The most common type of surgery for enlarged prostate without cancer (transurethral resection of the prostate, or TURP) does not usually cause impotence. In this surgery the prostate is reduced in size and removed through the urethra.

Multiple sclerosis is a disease of the nerves affecting the brain and spinal cord. It can cause impotence, as can spinal cord injuries that damage the nerves that control erection.

The Search Continues: Psychological Causes

"In my head? No way!" Of course not. No man wants to think that his failure to have an erection is psychological. However, stress and other psychological factors can certainly contribute to erection problems. About 30 percent of cases in some studies were found to be from psychological causes. Stress may aggravate another condition causing impotence. For example, when stress causes blood pressure to shoot up, the antihypertensive medication causes impotence. Yet, there are some cases when the best treatment is psychological counseling to correct the problem.

Psychological causes are treatable, so it is important not to ignore this possibility if no other causes are found. Plus, there are steps that you can take on your own. For example, learning a few stress management skills can greatly reduce the way you react to stressful situations. You may need only to reduce your stress to solve your erection problem.

A Depressed Libido

Depression is another cause of erectile dysfunction. Up to 90 percent of depressed men suffer from some type of erection problem. In the past, many doctors failed to recognize depression in male patients and often treated them with anxiety medications or told them to reduce their stress. In today's tumultuous corporate world, the rate of depression is rising faster among men than women, with more successful professional men in their thirties and forties reporting having this problem.

Which Came First?

Still, with depression there is the question of what causes the impotence—the depression or the antidepressants used to treat it. While specialists claim a success rate of up to 90 percent using a combination of medications (Paxil, Zoloft, or Prozac) along with behavioral psychotherapy, it's important to know the side effects of the medicine your doctor prescribes many antidepressants cause a decrease of libido.

If you find yourself experiencing sadness, depression, anger, or chronic stress, it may be helpful to consider evaluation by a clinical psychologist, psychiatrist, or sex therapist.

New Hope for a New Millennium

It is now possible to be sexually active your entire life. If you have put off talking with your doctor—or even your loved one—about a problem with impotence, do it today.

As you will learn later in this book, there are medications, such as Viagra, vacuum devices, injections, and surgical treatments that can cure impotence in most cases. All of these are proven to help return the enjoyment of sexual activity to men and their partners.

If you gain just one fact from this book, we want you to know that with the treatments available today, almost every man can be helped to overcome erectile dysfunction. Keep reading to find the right therapy to help you become sexually active once more.

PART I

The Real Facts About Impotence

Chapter 1

GET THE SCOOP ON...
Sexual stimulation starts in the brain ▪ Stress and fatigue can cause erectile difficulties ▪ Aging and sexual performance ▪ Normal bodily changes that occur with age ▪ Prostate concerns and aging

A Look at the Male Anatomy

Before we discuss the latest treatment choices for impotence, or erectile dysfunction, it is important to understand its causes.

Every man is different. The specific medication or treatment that works for a family member, friend, or the convincing actor on the "herbal cure for impotence" commercial may not be the correct one for you. In fact, it is difficult to really understand erectile dysfunction without a clear and thorough appreciation of the physiology of the male anatomy.

Many common diseases, medications, certain surgeries, and such life interruptions as stress, anxiety, or depression can affect your ability to achieve and maintain an erection. Even being overly tired or excessive worries can cause erectile difficulties.

Few people realize that having a natural erection is a complex process. While sensations of sexual arousal begin in the brain, obstructions between the brain and the penis can render the erection unsatisfactory. For example, some men might have

> "Just because a man has an occasional problem with having an erection does not mean it will develop into a chronic condition.—Mike, 49, urologist"

trouble getting any type of erection. Others may complain of getting only a partial erection, making it difficult to sustain penetration. Still other men may not be able to keep the erection and seek help because it is no longer predictable.

No matter what type of erectile dysfunction you experience, you will be relieved to know that for most men, treatment is now available. However, before we discuss the latest treatment methods, let's review the male anatomy, along with problems that may interrupt normal functioning of the male genitalia.

Checking Out the Male Genitalia

The penis is divided into two external parts (see Figure 1.1). Within the body of the penis are three sections:

- The corpus spongiosum penis, which contains the urethra, through which urine passes from the bladder.
- Two corpora cavernosum, sometimes called "erection chambers," are responsible for causing an erection.
- The glans penis is the end portion of the penis and is made up of the expansion of the corpus spongiosum.

FIGURE 1.1: LINE ART OF PENIS

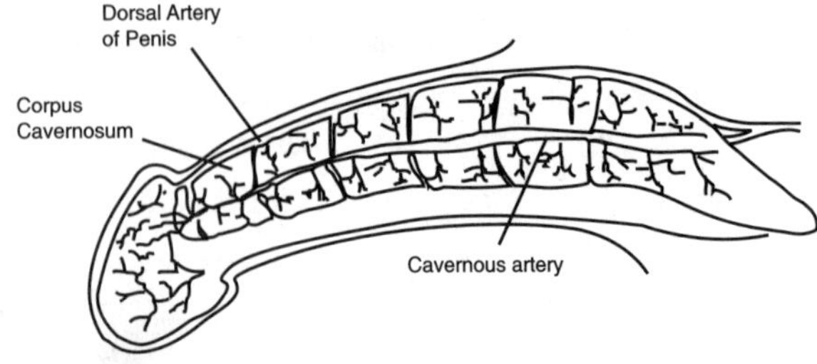

Between each of the two corpora cavernosum, there is a permeable partition that allows blood to travel from one corpora cavernosum to the other. For those with erectile dysfunction, this also allows medication injected in one side to travel to the other.

The root of the penis and surrounding tissue are supported by a host of muscles and ligaments and are attached by other tissue to the pubic bone. Arteries from the pelvis supply blood to the penis, while arteries in each of the corpora cavernosum supply blood for erections. The dorsal artery travels along the upper surface of the penis to supply the glans penis (see Figure 1.2).

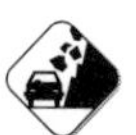

Watch Out!
Your mind has a very powerful influence over your sexual performance. Just worrying about your ability to perform sexually can sabotage your erections.

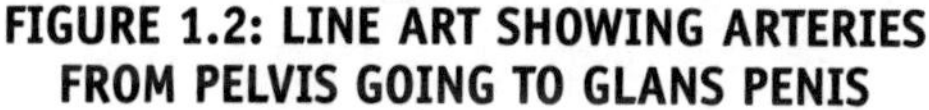

FIGURE 1.2: LINE ART SHOWING ARTERIES FROM PELVIS GOING TO GLANS PENIS

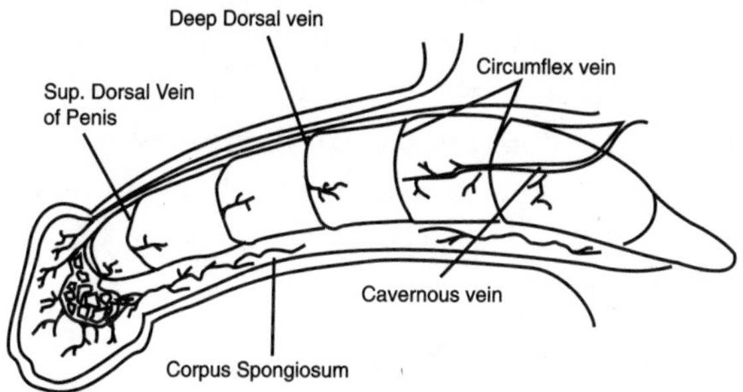

The veins that drain the blood away from the penis combine to join larger veins in the pelvis and carry the blood back toward the heart. Nerve impulses to the penis that cause erections originate from the lower portion of the spinal cord.

How an erection begins

When you are sexually aroused, your brain sends signals to the nerves in the penis. Touch or direct sensory contact can also stimulate these penile nerves. These nerve impulses travel to the two corpora cavernosum, causing the penile arteries to expand and an increase in blood flow to the penis. As the two "erection chambers" fill with blood, this causes pressure on the smaller veins that take blood away from the penis. These spaces change from the low volume of blood normally present to a high volume of blood that makes the penis hard and erect. As a result of more blood flowing in from the arteries and less blood flowing out through the smaller veins, the erection occurs.

Researchers have found that the penile nerves produce *nitric oxide,* the chemical "messenger" that allows an erection. Nitric oxide causes the blood vessels to relax in the corpora cavernosum. When the spaces containing blood relax, they become filled with blood and the erection occurs.

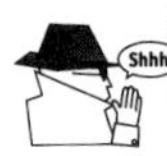

Unofficially... Medications such as Viagra help stimulate erections by increasing the amount of nitric oxide in the blood.

The erection diminishes when the spaces that contain blood in the corpora cavernosum become smaller, as the muscles and arteries contract. Likewise, the veins that carry blood out of the penis become less compressed, allowing more blood to flow away from the penis.

An "un-nerving" problem

Most people assume that an erection is a natural male function; just as many people are shocked when there is a problem. Yet any physical or emotional factor that affects a man's arteries, veins, nerves, or hormones can deactivate an erection. For example, erection problems can occur if nerve impulses are prevented from reaching the penis. These nerve problems can occur after injuries, in diseases such as diabetes and multiple sclerosis, and with other common medical problems.

Narrowed arteries can also cause erection problems by impeding blood flow to the penis. This common problem is frequently associated with aging. If the veins don't close off effectively, the blood cannot stay in the penis long enough to cause the erection.

Your doctor can measure penile blood pressure to assess blood flow to the penis. A more accurate ultrasound test can measure the quality of the arterial blood flow into the penis. Other tests can ascertain whether the small veins that carry blood out of the penis close off properly during erection. There are also tests for analyzing nerve problems, but accurate testing can be complicated and is not done very often. In some cases, however, it may be worth the trouble to pinpoint problems with the nerves leading to the penis or in the spinal cord. Your doctor can guide you to a neurologist or a clinic that specializes in this testing. All of these tests will be discussed in chapter 2.

Lack of desire

"Libido" means sexual desire, and, in men, testosterone is the major player with libido. With loss of libido, men have less desire for sexual activity and usually have fewer sexual fantasies.

There may be many reasons for loss of libido in men. Your doctor can determine if there are specific medical problems causing a loss of desire. One of the most common and easily treatable causes is a low level of testosterone. If this is found to be the cause, treatment to increase testosterone can restore libido. Testosterone levels normally decrease as men age. This decline can begin in the twenties, continues throughout a man's life, and increases especially after age 60. However, despite the lower levels, most men usually retain enough testosterone effect to render treatment unnecessary.

Psychological problems such as depression may bring a loss of sexual desire. Researchers found 75 percent of depressed people lose sex drive. Most of these people, however, reported the return of normal libido after treatment for their depression. Because some antidepressants can actually contribute to loss of libido, it is important to be aware of these possible side effects. In fact, most of the medications commonly used to treat depression have been linked to loss of libido or erectile dysfunction. Wellbutrin and Serzone, however, are two drugs that are not usually associated with loss of libido. In fact, some patients report an increase of libido when using the antidepressant Wellbutrin.

> "I had difficulty maintaining an erection for a period when I was first married. I was only 29 years old at the time, and this frightened me. I knew my manhood was gone. You can imagine my relief when I read the side effect of erectile dysfunction for some stomach remedy my doctor had prescribed. Once I was able to stop the stomach medication, my impotency problem ended.—Sam, 35, banker"

Problems in the relationship with the partner can show up as loss of desire, and anger can actually cause erectile dysfunction. In these cases, counseling may solve the problem of loss of sexual desire.

People who have suffered previous sexual abuse may have problems with libido. Counseling by a psychologist or psychiatrist is the most effective way to resolve this limitation on sexual desire.

Some religious beliefs may make it difficult or unacceptable to maintain libido because of guilt or other factors. Previous feelings of rejection by a sexual partner and the anxiety created by fear of failure in sexual activities (i.e., performance anxiety) may lower libido as a form of self-protection against further rejection or failure. Counseling can help to correct this cause of loss of libido.

The embarrassment of erectile dysfunction can also lead to a loss of sexual desire. In fact, many men manage their failure to have an erection by avoiding sexual activity altogether. Performance anxiety may overshadow other activities, as well. Once this problem is treated, it is common for the libido to return to normal. The lifting of anxiety and stress may even bring a dramatic increase in libido.

Medical problems such as chronic pain, heart disease, kidney disease, liver disease, lung disease, and drug and alcohol problems can cause fatigue, depression, and loss of libido. Treatment of the underlying medical problem may help return libido to normal levels.

Medications used for hypertension, tranquilizers, and antidepressants can also lower libido.

A simple difference in levels of desire may make one partner's level appear to be abnormally low. Open discussion may solve this perceived libido problem. Keep in mind as well that day to day, normal variations in libido are common. A brief change does not necessarily mean that your libido has changed forever.

Bright Idea
If you are taking a drug that may affect sexual function and libido, check with your doctor if you feel an uncomfortable drop in libido.

The Purpose of the Ejaculation Reflex

It's important to understand that ejaculation has nothing to do with having an erection. Many men who experience erectile dysfunction have no problem achieving orgasm and ejaculation with a soft penis.

The ejaculation reflex allows for delivery of the sperm during the climax in sexual intercourse. Nerve messages from the brain and from the nerves of the penis trigger the nerve impulses that cause contraction of the passages leading from the testicles. The sperm and fluid from the passages travel to the urethra, but are not allowed to go backward into the bladder because the muscles at the bladder neck constrict and close it off. The release of the sperm and fluid and the accompanying feelings are the *orgasm.* At this moment, the muscles around the urethra contract to ensure ejaculation of the fluid and sperm.

Premature ejaculation—a common problem

Premature ejaculation is the most common type of ejaculation problem. This may have a different meaning to each couple and has no specific definition accepted by everyone. To most people, premature or early ejaculation can simply mean an ejaculation that occurs earlier than desired.

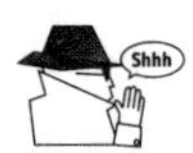

Unofficially... An estimated 15 percent of all men experience loss of libido at some time in their lives.

Many factors contribute to premature ejaculation

If the time to ejaculation is shorter than desired for satisfaction, then it can be called premature. This may happen on every occasion, or it can be a random event. High levels of stress and anxiety can aggravate premature ejaculation. Some researchers feel that premature ejaculation is a result of mainly psychological causes. However, some medications can treat premature ejaculation, which raises the possibility of physiological causes as well.

If you have a problem with premature ejaculation, try some of the following "self-help" tips:

- Enjoy your partner without focusing on your sexual performance.
- Use a strong, thicker condom that will lessen sensitivity.

- Try "squeeze therapy." As the ejaculation approaches, squeeze the head of your penis with your hand. Wait patiently while the response passes, then continue.
- Remember that practice makes perfect! Increase the frequency of your ejaculations to gain control.
- Ask your doctor for a referral to a sex therapist.

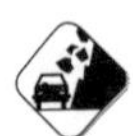

Watch Out!
A steady diet of hamburgers, french fries, and other high-fat foods might hinder your sexual pleasure. A study at the University of Utah found that fat-laden meals may curb the production of testosterone, the hormone that pumps up your sexual appetite.

Changes Associated with Aging

You can live on nutritional powershakes and pump iron for hours each day, but no one escapes the changes that come with age. Our bodies change with age, and it is important that these changes not be interpreted as abnormal or as a sign of disease.

Some changes, however, are less welcome than others, especially those that remind us that our bodies are aging (wrinkles, gray hair, a spreading waistline). Yet once we allow ourselves to accept that these changes cannot be avoided, we can manage them and keep them from limiting us.

Many of the changes of healthy aging, such as balding or the pull of gravity, do not by themselves create problems. They can, however, create anxiety *if* we allow ourselves to think they mean less activity, poor health, and, finally, death.

Changes in appearance

Healthy aging occurs at different rates in different people. Just as one child may mature earlier than another, adults can age differently.

After age 30, a decrease in the number of pigment cells result in changes in the skin. These cells allow tanning, so the ability to tan evenly may decrease with the cells. Harmless spots—th

remnants of these pigment cells—may appear. Skin may become thinner and bruise more easily. Changes in the fibers and thickness of the skin can also result in wrinkles and looser skin, especially in the face and neck.

Between the ages of 35 to 45, a build-up of more fat deposits may cause the size of the abdomen to gradually increase, even though total body weight may not. After the age of 40, some of the fat tissue under the skin may disappear and the spine, shoulder blades, and facial bones may become more apparent.

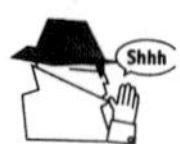

Unofficially... More than half the population over age 50 has some gray hair.

Gray hair is another sign of aging. It is the result of loss of pigment cells that give hair its color. Graying is usually gradual and may begin as early as age 20. More than half the population of the United States over age 50 has some gray hair. Thinning hair is another common change in aging men and women, although graying usually precedes it. In men, hair loss usually begins in the front of the scalp and gradually extends to cover the crown. Men usually do not lose hair along the fringe of the scalp. In fact, this hair is usually a great source for transplanting to other areas where hair has thinned. Loss of auxiliary hair is also common after age 60; pubic hair, underarm hair, and hair on the arms and legs may also decrease with age.

As the hair on your scalp thins, you may find new hair appearing elsewhere on your body. This hair is dark and short and may appear in "unwanted" places, over the ears, in the nose, or as thicker eyebrows. Inasmuch as these changes are considered unsightly by society's fashion standards, they are not signs of underlying diseases; they are normal changes of maturity.

TABLE 1.1: COMMON CHANGES IN MALES ASSOCIATED WITH AGING

Thirties	The number of pigment cells in the skin drops, making it harder to tan evenly. Hair on the scalp may begin to gray or thin. Brighter lights help vision as the size of the pupils becomes smaller. Frequent sex is still possible, as in the 20s. Level of testosterone may gradually decrease.
Forties	Body weight may increase. Wrinkles start on the forehead, near the corners of the eyes, or around the lips. Skin becomes more susceptible to damage from prolonged sun exposure. Gum disease becomes more prevalent, allowing tooth decay. Reading glasses may be needed.
Fifties	More than half of people have some gray hair on the scalp after age 50. It may take longer to achieve erection, and testosterone levels may drop. The prostate enlarges and studies show that 25 percent of men notice a decrease in the force of the urine stream by age 55.
Sixties and beyond	It may take up to two or three times longer to achieve erection, although studies show that 70 to 80 percent of couples are sexually active at age 68. Average weight levels off between 65 and 75, then gradually declines. Height drops about $^1/_2$ inch each 20 years after maturity. Fat tissue under the skin of the face decreases, making bones appear more prominent. Testosterone levels may drop at a faster rate.

Changes in sexual performance

Comprehensive research has found it common for men over age 50 to require longer periods of excitement to achieve full erection. This is not necessarily related to any health problem. Also, while it may take a little longer to experience full sexual pleasure, it definitely does not lessen the excitement you will feel. Think about it. While you may not run a mile as fast as you did at age 18, perhaps you now find more pleasure in the journey, noticing the trees and flowers along the way. As you age, it may take you longer to reach an erection, but this is *not* impotence. You can still enjoy sexual pleasure no matter what your age. You cannot wear out your penis!

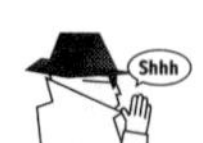

Unofficially... Your weight increases as you age, and usually peaks between ages 40 and 60. Your weight will begin to level off between ages 65 and 75, then gradually decline.

Instead of being surprised by sexual changes that occur with age, knowing ahead of time that these changes will occur can save you a great deal of stress and anxiety. In fact, awareness of these changes can reduce your anxiety, which can by itself disrupt your erection. Common sexual changes that occur with age include:

- Taking longer to achieve erection.
- An erection that is less hard than when you were younger.
- Increasing delays in orgasm and ejaculation.
- Less force in ejaculation.
- A decrease in the amount of fluid during ejaculation.
- Erection easily lost after orgasm.
- Difficulty regaining erection after orgasm.

Most researchers agree that aging does not have to mean an end to sexual activity, and that the need for physical contact continues throughout our entire life. In fact, most men and women who communicate openly about their feelings adjust quite well to the bodily changes that accompany age. Some researchers have found that even at age 68, more than 70 percent of couples remain sexually active. Others have reported that more than 80 percent of couples over age 60 were sexually active, and at least half had regular sexual activity.

Prostate Concerns and Aging

As men age, the prostate gland is guaranteed to almost always increase in size. The prostate gland is situated at the base of the bladder, near the urethra, which is the tube that carries urine out of the bladder through the penis (see Figure 1.3). The prostate produces fluid that is mixed with sperm.

The first changes commonly start by around age 35 with some increase in size and number of the glands. Over half of men have symptoms of prostate enlargement by age 69, and almost every man develops the condition eventually.

> “I got married for the second time at the age of 76, and my new bride was 75. We feel like we are still on our honeymoon and enjoy being sexually intimate with the help of an injected drug for erectile dysfunction.—Mac, 79, retired”

What you might feel

Prostate enlargement is very gradual. The symptoms can occur either from blockage of the flow of urine from the bladder or from irritation of the bladder (see Figure 1.3). Blockage occurs when the enlarged prostate gland compresses the urethra, which carries the urine. This causes the size and force of the urine stream to become smaller. Compression against the urethra also means that more pressure is now needed for urine to pass, and it takes longer to start the flow of urine. Difficulty maintaining the higher pressure may also cause an intermittent flow of urine—waiting periods during urination—until the bladder has completely emptied. There may be some dribbling at the very end of urination.

Frequency of urination often increases when the prostate becomes enlarged. The bladder may not empty completely, as just discussed, so it must empty more often. Also, prostate enlargement irritates the bladder and causes more frequent emptying. These symptoms are more common at night when we do not consciously ignore the sensations. At night the tightness of the muscles that control the release of urine is usually less, which adds to the frequency.

Medications can aggravate any of the above symptoms. For example, antihistamines can slow the control of the release of urine.

FIGURE 1.3: LINE ART SHOWING NORMAL MALE URINARY TRACT

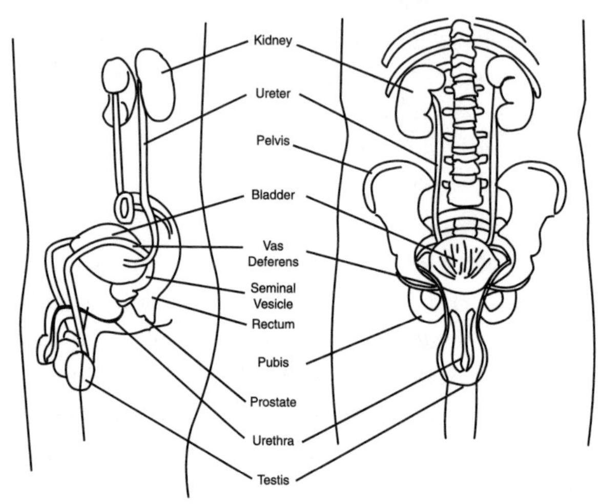

Medications that successfully treat an enlarged prostate

There are a few simple questions that specialists have developed that can give a good idea as to whether further treatment might be needed for an enlarged prostate. After a careful history and physical examination, your doctor will guide you as to the best treatment.

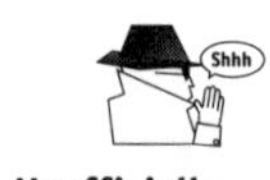

Unofficially... According to Masters and Johnson, at least 25 to 30 percent of people in their 60s have intercourse at least weekly.

Every man's greatest fear

The incidence of prostate cancer is rare before age 40, then gradually increases with age (see Table 2.3). The good news is that prostate cancer can be controlled if diagnosed in time, so it is important to know the facts. Early testing is the key to effective treatment.

There are usually no symptoms of early prostate cancer, which is when you would want to make the diagnosis. Blockage of urine flow, blood in the urine, or problems controlling urination may indicate the cancer is in later stages. Usually by the time these symptoms are present, it may be too late. A PSA (prostate-specific antigen) blood test, however, may provide early detection.

The answer is an examination by your doctor with routine yearly testing of the prostate by rectal examination and PSA blood test. If a nodule or other irregularity is found in the prostate, then your doctor may ask you to see a urologist to decide whether a biopsy is necessary. The PSA blood test is used to find prostate cancer at an early stage.

Watch Out!
If you have a family member with prostate cancer, you may be at higher than average risk, especially if he was affected when in his forties or fifties.

Some experts feel that the value of the PSA test can be increased if age is taken into account, with a slight increase in PSA levels allowable in men age 70 to 79. (A normal test ranges from 0 to 4.0 ng/ml.) Also, your doctor can tell by repeating the PSA test in six to 12 months whether the chances are high enough for cancer to warrant biopsy.

There is more than one type of PSA in the blood. Your doctor can determine if an elevated PSA is attributable to *free* PSA, which is associated with benign prostate enlargement, or to *bound or complex* PSA, which is more commonly associated with prostate cancer.

There are some arguments about the use of the PSA test since it can result in biopsies in patients who don't have prostate cancer. On the other hand, it is in this group of patients that prostate cancer in its earliest and most treatable and curable stages may be found. If you are a man over age 50, you should have a yearly PSA and prostate examination. If you are an African–American man or have a family history of prostate cancer, you might consider beginning testing at around age 40.

Knowledge Is Crucial

"I can understand how an erection happens, but how is this information going to help me solve my problem with impotence?" We know that the main reason you opened this book is not to read about the functioning of the male genitalia. However, it has long been recognized that when many men suffering from erectile dysfunction are given a diagnosis, much of their anxiety and distress results from a *lack of knowledge* about their particular problem. Not only are they frightened from the inability to perform sexually, but they are also uneasy about what lies ahead. The fear can in fact be overwhelming.

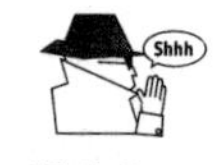

Unofficially... In the United States, African-Americans are affected by prostate cancer 50 percent more than whites.

The information in this book, along with an acute awareness of how your body functions and your specific erectile problem, will help you to regain control of your sexual function. This includes following any medication regime your doctor may prescribe, exercising regularly, eating nutritional foods, getting enough sleep, and trying alternative therapies to de-stress your body. In doing so, you will start on the path to total health, which, no matter what your age, will greatly enhance your quality of life and sexual pleasure.

Just the Facts

- Understanding how the male body works is the first step to understanding impotence.
- Stress, overwork, performance anxiety, and prescription medications can all cause impotence.
- Changes associated with aging do not have to mean an end to sexual activity.
- Prostate cancer can be cured with early diagnosis and treatment.

Chapter 2

GET THE SCOOP ON...

A visit to your doctor is the first step toward ending erectile dysfunction ▪ Impotence problems that require a specialist ▪ Choosing a doctor with whom you feel comfortable ▪ How tests for diagnosing impotence could also save your life

Getting Some Answers

It's not easy to talk about impotence. Maybe even buying or reading this book makes you feel uncomfortable or self-conscious. Nonetheless, if you suffer from impotence, the sooner you discuss it with your partner and your doctor, the sooner you can return to a fulfilling sexual relationship. With the treatments now available, including use of the drug Viagra, most men can quickly and easily reverse this condition and feel sexually confident again.

For any man who suffers with impotence, regaining control starts when you call your doctor, seek an accurate diagnosis, adhere to the treatment your doctor prescribes, and report any abnormal symptoms.

But you can't solve your erectile problem if you don't *call your doctor.* Taking this step will put you back in control of your life and your sexual prowess!

Working with Your Doctor

Your doctor plays the first significant role in reversing of your erectile dysfunction. Not only does he or she serve as the one who can accurately diagnose and prescribe treatment, this healthcare professional knows how impotence can affect you and your partner, and may become a close, dependable friend to talk to when concerns turn into ongoing worries and anxieties. Many marriages and long-term relationships have been destroyed because of impotence; having someone to talk to may just save yours.

Your doctor is thus essential to solving your problem with impotence. Because of the increasingly common managed care system, however, finding the right person to diagnose and treat impotence properly and cost-effectively is not always easy. The following suggestions may help.

Talk to your primary care physician

If you have a primary care physician, make sure that he is fully aware of your medical history. If you don't have a primary care physician, engage one you can trust to take responsibility for your overall healthcare. This general practitioner or internist is your primary care doctor and is better able to assess your problems and make the necessary referrals to a specialist—a urologist, cardiologist, endocrinologist, or psychologist—if you need further treatment or special care for a secondary problem such as prostate disease, heart disease, diabetes, or depression.

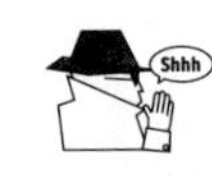

Unofficially... What is impotence again? Erectile dysfunction, or impotence, is defined as an inability to obtain and/or maintain an erection more than 20 percent of the time. This means that one out of five erections just don't work as well as they should.

Evaluate your need for a specialist

After selecting a primary care physician, many men question whether they also need a specialist. As a rule, if your response to treatment is unsatisfactory, you might consider talking with a specialist. Especially when coexisting illnesses and/or treatments complicate the treatment of erectile dysfunction, you should consult with a specialist in that field.

Be aware that problems may occur when you have more than one doctor administering treatment. Unless effective communication takes place between the physicians, you might find yourself in a precarious situation as far as your health is concerned. For example, your cardiologist may prescribe antihypertensives (medications for high blood pressure), which have erectile dysfunction as a main side effect. In turn, your high blood pressure medicine could render your impotence treatment ineffective, and leave your primary physician wondering why his treatment isn't working. Unless your doctors are aware of all diagnoses and medications, you will have difficulty getting to the root of your problem.

While both doctors may be working to keep you well, it is important to have one doctor who knows all about you—your condition, your symptoms, your treatment plan, and the specific medications you are taking. Keeping each doctor informed of all details of your treatment, including changes in medications, can only speed your recovery. Specialists who treat impotence include:

- Cardiologist: a doctor who specializes in the diagnosis and treatment of disorders of the heart and blood vessels.
- Endocrinologist: a doctor who specializes in the study of the internal or hormonal secretions and how they act in the body.

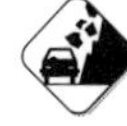

Watch Out!
Men who have a congenital venous leak never experience really hard erections. This condition occurs when the venous drainage system in the penis does not shut down properly during sexual arousal, resulting in blood draining from the penis, limiting full erection. This problem can usually be corrected without surgery.

- Neurologist: a doctor who specializes in the diagnosis and treatment of disorders of the neuromuscular system, specifically the nerves and muscles.
- Internist: a doctor who specializes in internal medicine, the study of diseases in adults.
- Primary care physician: a doctor who is a general practitioner, a family practice doctor, or an internist.
- Psychiatrist: a doctor who specializes in the treatment of mental disorders.
- Psychologist: a doctor or professional who specializes in the study of the behavior of humans and related mental and physical processes.
- Urologist: a doctor who specializes in diseases and problems of the genitourinary tract, which includes the kidneys, adrenal glands, bladder, prostate gland, testicles, and related structures.

Check age, sex, and credentials

In choosing a healthcare professional, some people ask friends for recommendations, check the physician's credentials, or call the local hospital for referrals. In this age of managed care, you will also need to check the list of doctors who will accept your insurance provider.

Perhaps one of the most important steps to take when selecting a healthcare professional is to know yourself, including your personal preferences. Do you feel more comfortable with a man or a woman? Should your physician be older than you, the same age, or younger? Do you have a preference as to educational background? These questions are important to consider when making your appointment.

Ask the following questions as you go through the process of choosing a physician.

- Is the doctor board certified? This means that the doctor passed a standard exam given by the governing board in his or her specialty.
- Where did the doctor go to medical school? Your local medical society can provide this information.
- Is the doctor involved in any academic pursuits, such as teaching, writing, or research? This doctor may be more up-to-date in the latest developments in his or her field.
- Where does your doctor have hospital privileges, and where are these hospitals located? Some doctors may not admit patients to certain hospitals, and this is an important consideration for those with chronic health problems.

Plan a consultation

Plan an initial consultation with the doctor during which you can get to know each other. This will include a detailed interview and physical examination. During this initial interview ask questions as to the preferred methods of treatment. Is he or she current in using the latest methods of treatment?

Open patient/physician communication is important if you are to receive not only the highest quality of care, but also comfort you'll need during anxious moments. Does the physician appear to relate well to people? Do you feel at ease in talking with the doctor? Are your questions answered?

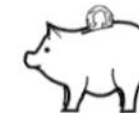

Moneysaver
Make sure the doctor you choose accepts your particular type of health insurance. If not, you will be paying out-of-pocket for all healthcare.

Your physician needs to be accessible. When you have a more serious illness, popularity is not important, but availability is. Make sure your doctor is not only a skilled physician, but one who is also available and attentive to your personal needs. Does the doctor allow ample time with you so that quality care is received? Are your questions answered clearly, and are necessary tests made?

Check on office hours, and make sure these fit with your daily schedule. How is payment made? What insurance providers are accepted? Ask for information about emergency availability and charges. Is your doctor always on call or are other doctors sharing responsibility? Even the receptionist's responses help you decide if this is the right office. The support staff will be the ones who help you most with prescriptions, obtaining necessary lab work, x-rays, and making appointments with hospitals or other professional services.

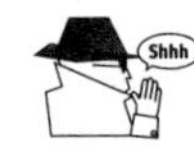

Unofficially... Before Viagra, most men were treated by external vacuum therapy, penile injection, implant surgery, or intraurethral pellet implantation. Estimates of treatments prescribed annually include 150,000 vacuum devices, 700,000 penile injections, and 21,000 penile implants.

And, let's not forget that with the increased demands on our healthcare system, mistakes can be made. Medical errors can result from under-testing, (not enough tests to make a correct evaluation), incorrect testing, or even over-testing (far more tests than necessary). Clearly, the only way to guard against this is to be assertive and knowledgeable as you take responsibility for your health.

Changes in medical coverage may mean that the doctor you now see will not be the one you see in a year or two. This makes it even more important to understand your particular problem fully, stay abreast of treatment methods, and fully follow the management plan discussed in this book.

Impotence and Your Medical History

If you are experiencing erectile problems, your doctor needs to know because your impotence may be a symptom of some other, more serious disease. For example, erectile dysfunction is sometimes an early symptom of diabetes. Knowing this, your doctor can test for diabetes. Nerve damage can also cause erectile dysfunction, as can heart problems. A good doctor will look into each of these areas to make sure nothing more serious is taking place.

Some specific questions will help your doctor understand your impotence problem and recommend a treatment plan that really works. Let your doctor know that finding a solution to your erection problem is important to you. In some cases, you may consider taking your spouse with you to the appointment, although this is not necessary. Do this if you feel more comfortable as a couple, since it is a "couple's issue."

Watch Out!
While you may not be surprised that stress can cause elevated blood pressure, did you know that stress can negatively affect an erection? When you are stressed, the blood in your body moves into your muscles, helping you to get ready for the "fight or flight" reaction. This means that the nervous system moves blood needed for an erection away from the penis.

Getting to the root of your problem

As your doctor evaluates your situation and takes your personal medical history, he will ask specific questions to pinpoint the root cause of your erectile dysfunction. Some commonly asked questions include:

- Is the problem occasional or chronic (long-term)?
- Do you worry about having the problem even before it occurs?
- Do you use any medications?
- Do you drink alcohol? How much do you drink?

- Do you smoke cigarettes? How long have you smoked?
- Do you have peripheral vascular disease (hardening of the arteries, especially in the legs)?
- Does your family have a history of high blood pressure?
- Do you have a family history of diabetes?
- Do you have a history of depression?
- Have you had any past surgeries?
- Have you had any injuries to the groin area?
- What specific medical problems have you had that were treated with medication or surgery?
- Do you have erections at night during sleep?
- Do you have erections upon awakening in the mornings?
- When was the last time you had a normal erection?
- When was the last time you had sexual intercourse?
- Are your erections painful?
- Is your penis bent when erect?
- Do you worry that you will not be able to have an erection when needed?
- Do you worry that you will never again be able to have an erection?

Uncovering hidden stressors

We're sure it's no news to you that your mind and body are interconnected to an extent far surpassing previous assumptions, and physical health and emotional well-being are closely linked. Through scientific tests we also know that stress can literally wreck your health. In today's pressured society, chronic stress persists for days, weeks, or even months, tearing at your mind, body, and spirit. Stress also increases your body's production of *catecholamines (epinephrine and non-epinephrine)*, which inhibit erections.

Your doctor will ask about the stress in your life and will check to see if you are experiencing too much stress. See Table 2.1 for a list of common symptoms of stress.

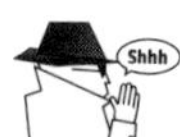

Unofficially... At least four in ten of all adults suffer adverse health effects from stress, and as many as nine in ten of all visits to doctors' offices are for stress-related complaints, according to the American Psychological Association.

TABLE 2.1: COMMON SYMPTOMS OF STRESS

Anger	Anxiety	Apathy	Chest pain or tightness
Back pain	Colitis	Depression	Heart palpitations
Headaches	Hives	Irritable bowel syndrome (IBS)	Impotence
Inability to relax	Inability to concentrate	Insomnia	Mood swings
Loss of sexual desire	Loss of sexual function	Neck pain	No energy
Rapid pulse	Rashes	Short temper	Short-term memory loss

Stress has also been linked to an increased risk of the following diseases and ailments:

- Allergies, asthma, and hay fever
- Backaches
- Cancer
- Heart disease
- High blood pressure
- Migraine headaches
- Stroke
- TMJ (temporomandibular joint) syndrome
- Tension headaches
- Peptic ulcer disease

The stress in your life can come from marital problems, work-related problems, fear of performance failure in sexual activities, or numerous other areas. Your doctor will need to ask many questions, but this doesn't mean that he is trying to pry into your personal life. The more he knows, the better able he will be to find a solution to your problem. Many times a doctor can help you unravel specific stumbling blocks in your relationships with others or at work and help you learn how to change these into stepping stones.

Tell your doctor what you expect your treatment to accomplish, so that the specific problems that bother you are addressed by the treatment prescribed.

Undergoing the Physical Examination

Once your doctor has discussed your problem, you'll have a physical exam to see if your erectile dysfunction is being caused by some other problem.

The basic physical

During your general examination, your doctor can check for certain medical problems that could be creating your erectile difficulties. For example, peripheral vascular disease in the legs impedes circulation and may indicate arterial blockage, which can cause erection problems. Other examinations include a rectal exam of the prostate. The nerve supply to the area can also be checked during this examination. Your doctor can also tell by examination whether there are any other physical problems involving the penis or testicles that can affect erection. These examinations are quick and painless. Try to limit your anxiety over this part of the examination, because it will greatly help to solve your erection problem as quickly and effectively as possible.

Laboratory tests may reveal serious problems

Some laboratory tests are needed to be sure no other medical problems are present that are contributing to the erection problem. For example, an accurate assessment of testosterone levels may be needed. While it is rare that low testosterone would affect your erections, the lower levels would affect your initial sexual desire or libido. Diabetes mellitus

TABLE 2.2: COMMONLY USED TESTS TO DIAGNOSE THE CAUSE OF IMPOTENCE

Assessment of circulation in the legs and feet.
Assessment of reflexes and nerves in the legs and feet.
Assessment of penile blood pressure to measure blood flow.
Evaluation of testicle size to assess hormone status.
Inspection of prostate through a rectal-prostate exam.
Laboratory tests (blood tests) to measure thyroid function, testosterone level, cholesterol level, and to check for diabetes.
Oral or written questionnaire to assess your levels of stress.

can be found by measuring the blood glucose. Problems with the thyroid gland, whether overactive or underactive, can aggravate erection dysfunction and are found mainly by blood tests.

Infections can aggravate erectile dysfunction, so urine tests can help discover these when present. Other medical problems can be found through a general medical evaluation with your primary care physician.

Other tests might be ordered to give specific information to your doctor on the arterial blood supply to the penis or to test the nerves or the veins. Or, you might be asked to take a test that measures erections during sleep. This test measures "nocturnal tumescence and rigidity" (NPTR). For the NPTR test, you will attach a pair of special gauges to your penis prior to falling asleep. Because normal men of all ages have erections during the dreaming (rapid eye movement or REM) stages of their sleep, the NPTR test will measure these erections. If no nocturnal erection occurs or if the erection is hampered, the cause of your erectile dysfunction is likely to be physical. Nonetheless, if you have a normal NPTR yet have erectile dysfunction during sexual intercourse, it may stem from a psychological cause.

Timesaver
A simple fasting blood glucose or blood glucose two hours after a meal or even a two-hour glucose tolerance test may save your life—as well as your erections. Make sure your doctor does one of these tests if diabetes is a concern or runs in your family. It will save great stress and takes little time.

Keep in mind that most of these tests may not be necessary, and you may be started on treatment the first visit.

A comprehensive health review

Depending on your sex, age, and personal health history, your doctor will also review risk factors for coronary heart disease, cancer, diabetes, and osteoporosis and discuss removal or control of these risk factors. Your doctor can also schedule hearing, eye, or dental examinations, a skin test for tuberculosis, as well as other necessary tests.

During your visit to the doctor, ask about necessary immunizations. Adults need a tetanus booster every 10 years. Ask about any other immunizations that are necessary for your situation.

If you're at high risk, you should have a colonoscopy at age 40. If you have a family member (father, mother, brother, sister) with colon cancer, you should have a colonoscopy every three to five years. Check with your doctor.

Selecting the Best Treatment

After the doctor's evaluation, your urologist (or sometimes your primary care doctor or internist) will make a plan to correct the erectile dysfunction. You may be given trials of medications. Before you start, be sure you understand when and how to take the medication and what the side effects might be. Your doctor will then check the effectiveness of the treatment and decide if other steps are needed.

TABLE 2.3:
THE MOST COMMON CAUSES OF IMPOTENCE

Diabetes	Neurologic impairment	Prescription medications
Pelvic injury	Psychological disorders	Peyronie's disease
Vascular disease	Hormonal imbalance	

Other choices in treatment may include medications inserted in the penis, a vacuum device to create an erection, or injections of medications into the penis. Another possible treatment is a gel that is applied to the penis. The medication in this gel is absorbed through the skin of the penis to stimulate erection. Surgery is also possible to correct some

Bright Idea
Brown Bag It. To make sure your doctor knows all your medications, vitamins, and supplements, pack them in a paper bag and take to your next doctor's visit. This will help him or her protect you against a drug interaction that may result in erectile dysfunction.

medical problems and can be considered when all other treatments fail. Penile prosthesis insertion, of course, requires surgery.

With the new medications available, it seems easy to choose one to cure erectile dysfunction. But a cure is not possible without first discovering the cause. Remember, 80 percent or more of cases are likely to have a physical cause, so correcting the underlying physical problem could also cure the erectile dysfunction.

TABLE 2.4: GUIDELINES FOR REGULAR EXAMINATIONS AND PREVENTIVE MEASURES FOR MEN

Examination	Frequency
Physical Exam	Every three years from age 20 to 39
	Every two years from age 40 to 49
	Every year after 50
Blood Pressure	Every year
Tuberculosis	Every five years from age 20 to 39
Blood and Urine Tests	Every three years from age 20 to 39
	Every two years from age 40 to 49
	Every year after age 50
Electrocardiogram	Every three to five years after age 50 or after age 30 if at high risk for heart attack
Rectal Exam	Every year after age 40
Tetanus Booster	Every 10 years
PSA Blood Test	Every year after 50, or every year after age 40 if at high risk of prostate disease.
Hemoccult	Every year after age 40.
Sigmoidoscopy	Every five years after 50 (check with your doctor).

Questions You May Have

After deciding to seek professional help to solve your erectile dysfunction, there are a number of questions that you will want to ask. These include:

- Ask about your risk factors so you can correct those over which you have control. This will allow you to prevent the most likely causes of serious illness and death—atherosclerosis (which causes heart attack), heart failure, stroke, and kidney failure.
- Ask about necessary tests for the most common kinds of cancer—prostate cancer, lung cancer, and colon cancer—and how to watch for melanoma and other skin cancers.
- Ask if your history or family history suggests any other specific health risks that should concern you.
- Ask about medications you are taking and the known side effects.

Just the Facts

- Consulting a physician is the first step toward curing impotence.
- Your medical history could hold the key to curing your erectile dysfunction.
- A physical examination will help you pin down the specific cause of your impotence.
- Laboratory tests (blood tests) can help find clues to your erectile dysfunction by measuring thyroid function, testosterone level, cholesterol level, and seeing if diabetes is present.
- Your doctor may relate your erectile dysfunction problem to diabetes, a hormonal imbalance, a neurologic impairment, pelvic injury, a common prescription medication, or to stress.

PART II

The Lowdown On Physical Causes

Chapter 3

GET THE SCOOP ON...

Testosterone, sexual desire, and erectile functioning ▪ Cortisol (the hormone secreted during times of high stress) and aging ▪ The intimate connection between the brain and body as it regulates how much testosterone is produced ▪ New theories on male menopause

The Reality of Aging

You're looking for the best car for your needs, wants, and money—but if the latter was no object, would your choices be different? Getting what will make you happy and not bust your budget is an art.

Let's face it. While most people think of only death and taxes as guaranteed certainties in life, there is another reality that we must also consider: we are all getting older. Past generations more readily accepted the steady decline of physical and mental functioning many still associate with aging. However, studies reveal that most people today continue to place a high value on being active and staying young.

Perhaps you can identify with the 53-year-old attorney who told his doctor, "I look and feel young and am at the top of my career, but I'm impotent and that makes me feel old and worn out." While the stumbling block of impotence used to put a damper on sexual relationships for millions of men aged forty and over, this does not have to be the case today. In fact, with open communication, a greater understanding of what causes impotence, and the newer treatments for this common problem, some men tell of feeling like they are again in their prime—mentally, physically, and sexually.

We *cannot* turn back the clock. Nonetheless, men of all ages can now reshape what it means to enjoy "prime time" performance at 30, 40, 50, 60... or even 80!

> "Testosterone, a male hormone, controls a host of bodily functions including growth, metabolism, sexual development, and reproduction. Too much or too little can lead to problems such as diabetes and weak bones.
> —Kim, research scientist, 41"

Changing Your Aging Attitude

No matter how many scientific breakthroughs give new insight into the causes of aging, no one has found a way to halt this natural process. To be honest, who would want to stop it, if they really could?

Think about it. Would you really want to be 18 again—and have to go through the many learning experiences to gain all the knowledge and wisdom you now have under your belt? Probably not. After all, healthy aging is the key to satisfaction and success. Not too many 18-year-olds are CEOs of large corporations or at the highest pinnacle in their respective careers.

Today, scientists are rewriting the rules of aging, and the prevailing opinion now holds that if a Galapagos turtle can live to be 152 years old, then maybe we can, too. Many researchers now believe that our life span need not be limited, and suggest that by taking responsibility for our health and lifestyle, we may slow down the aging process.

Think positive prevention

For years most of us have trusted science to determine our longevity. While many factors influence our health and life span, it seemed to be etched in stone that women outlived men, and if your parents died at an early age, you would too. While 66 years was the average life span in 1950, 75 years is the average today.

Healthy aging means using the positive aspects of your age, including expertise gained from life experiences, while you minimize negative aspects such as heart disease, cancer, diabetes, and other medical problems. In doing this, you may increase your life span as well as the number of years you are active and vital.

Taking a look at the most common problems of aging, such as osteoporosis (thinning of the bones), heart disease, or even cancer, it is amazing how a few simple preventative steps can protect against these causes of serious illness and death. For example, eating a high-calcium diet and exercising regularly can help keep your bones strong, even in your senior years. Keeping your blood pressure and cholesterol at normal levels, eating a low-fat, high complex carbohydrate diet, exercising, and managing your stress can help you prevent serious heart problems. Not smoking cigarettes can nearly eliminate lung cancer, and screening can control prostate and colon cancer. In most cases, these problems can be detected early enough that treatment will keep symptoms at bay.

Lifestyle plays a big role in aging

But what is the point of living to be 100 if you aren't healthy? The fact that you are reading this book is a good indicator that good health, prevention of disease, and quality of life are all important to you. Because of new breakthroughs in the early diagnosis and treatment of once-terminal diseases, the outlook for health in later years is remarkably better than in the past. In fact, most of us can coast to our mid-thirties on the virtue of good genes alone. But as we approach 40, our luck comes to a screeching halt. You see, there is a guaranteed time of awakening—

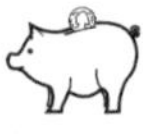

Moneysaver
Looking for an inexpensive way to decrease stress and increase immune function? Then take time to laugh frequently throughout your day. Not only will it help you live longer, it costs nothing! Studies show that a real belly laugh can increase antibodies that fight infection as well as decrease cortisol, a stress hormone that suppresses the immune system.

TABLE 3.1: HOLMES-RAHE SOCIAL READJUSTMENT SCALE

Life Events	Score
Death of spouse	100
Divorce	73
Marital separation from mate	65
Detention in jail, other institution	63
Death of a close family member	63
Major personal injury or illness	53
Marriage	50
Fired from work	47
Marital reconciliation	45
Retirement	45
Major change in the health or behavior of a family member	44
Sexual difficulties	39
Gaining a new family member (e.g., through birth, adoption, etc.)	39
Major business re-adjustment (e.g., merger, reorganization, bankruptcy)	39
Major change in financial status	38
Death of close friend	37
Change to different line of work	36
Major change in the number of arguments with spouse	35
Taking out a mortgage or loan for a major purchase	31
Foreclosure on a mortgage or loan	30
Major change in responsibilities at work	29
Son or daughter leaving home (e.g., marriage, attending college)	29
Trouble with in-laws	29
Outstanding personal achievement	28
Spouse beginning or ceasing to work outside the home	26
Beginning or ceasing formal schooling	26
Major change in living conditions	25
Revision of personal habits (e.g., dress, manners, associations, etc.)	24

Trouble with boss	23
Major change in working hours or conditions	20
Change in residence	20
Change to a new school	20
Major change in usual type and/or amount of recreation	19
Major change in church activities (e.g., a lot more or less than usual)	19
Major change in social activities (e.g., clubs, dancing, movies, visiting)	18
Taking out loan for a lesser purchase (e.g., for a car, TV, freezer, etc.)	17
Major change in sleeping habits	16
Major change in the number of family get-togethers	15
Major change in eating habits	15
Vacation	13
Christmas season	12
Minor violations of the law (e.g., traffic tickets, etc.)	11
TOTAL___________	

Less than 150 life change units = 30% chance of developing a stress-related illness
150-299 life change units = 50% chance of illness
Over 300 life change units = 80% chance of illness

usually during midlife—when the role of genetics subsides and lifestyle factors take over. Surprisingly, research concludes that only about 30 percent of the characteristics of aging are genetically based; the remaining 70 percent are determined by lifestyle. In fact, study after study now confirms that more than 85 percent of deaths are because of chronic conditions that can be prevented or alleviated by lifestyle changes.

Holding Back Age-Related Diseases

New breakthroughs in aging research may lead to innovative medical therapies to postpone age-related degenerative diseases by developing treatments for conditions ranging from heart disease and dementia to arthritis and wrinkles, and, yes, perhaps even to extend the human life span.

"I'm not worried about those diseases. I just feel old and tired." Many people complain of "feeling old," and for men, feeling out of sorts or "old" can put them at higher risk of erectile dysfunction. Yet what causes this "feeling," and can we change it? The answer may depend on your own lifestyle.

Comprehensive aging research now suggests that changes in cortisol secretion and decreased levels of sex steroids and growth hormone result in a cluster of symptoms such as low energy, perceptions of happiness, altered body composition, heart disease, and non-insulin-dependent diabetes. Some scientists refer to these changes as "premature aging processes" and suggest that psychosocial stressors, such as moving, losing a job, or losing a mate through divorce or death, as well as detrimental lifestyle habits such as alcohol consumption and smoking, are all involved in "premature aging."

Bright Idea
Every time you encounter stress, stop before thoughts escalate; breathe deeply to release physical tension; focus on the problem at hand and consider the cause of the stress; then choose how to deal with the stress.

The good news is that most of these stressors are controllable, meaning you can change your reaction to what happens in life—no matter how sudden or traumatic it may be.

Check out Table 3.1, and see how life's stressors may come back to haunt you in upcoming months. Circle the numbers that correspond to life events you've experienced this year, then add your score. Using the Holmes-Rahe social readjustment scale, see what chances you have of getting a stress-related illness in the near future. Keep in mind that while stress happens to all of us, we all have the ability to control our reaction to it.

Mind Over Midlife

The media attention recently given to menopause, has led some researchers to ask if men undergo a similar period. This period in life is often called "andropause" or "viropause," and refers to the loss of virility that often occurs in men in their 40s and 50s. During this time, a man's strength, sex drive, and peace of mind may take a nose dive. Some men come to believe that their best years are over, and tell of being extremely despondent or depressed. Others may make drastic changes like changing careers, buying a fast boat or sports car...or even leaving their wives and families for a younger partner.

Nonetheless, some researchers still claim that the male "midlife crisis" is purely pyschological. These scientists support their stand with reasonable explanations for the changes that men experience with aging.

According to some researchers, stress is a major contributor to the various symptoms of andropausal (male menopause) fatigue. Many researchers in the field of psychoneuroimmunology (the study of mind/body interplay) believe that the stress hormone cortisol increases in men during anticipatory stress, while the levels of total testosterone and LH (luteinizing hormone) decrease.

Stress also negatively affects our interest in sex. A man's sex drive is influenced by testosterone, which has daily and seasonal peaks.

Interestingly, hormonal problems, the result of endocrine or glandular disorders, account for only three percent of erectile failure. The testicles may produce too little testosterone, leading to a decrease in desire and sexual function. Also, brain or pituitary tumors may cause a buildup of prolactin, which in turn lowers testosterone levels and can lead to loss of libido.

The following bodily changes commonly occur in men between the ages of 40 and 70:

- Loss of 12 to 20 pounds of muscle.
- Loss of 15 percent of bone mass.
- Loss of two inches in height.
- Body metabolism slows down.
- Testicles shrink slightly.
- Sperm production declines.
- Thickened connective tissue in the prostate gland.
- Problems with urination and ejaculation.
- Functioning of the penis becomes sluggish.
- Erection chambers fill with connective tissue.
- Supporting arteries in the penis narrow.
- Subtle testosterone loss (about one percent per year after age 40 or 30 percent decline by age 70).

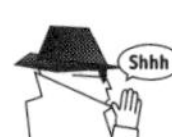

Unofficially... Between l998 and 2015, more than 11,000 Americans each day will turn 50. More than three million hit this milestone this year.

TABLE 3.2: SIGNS AND SYMPTOMS OF DECREASED TESTOSTERONE

Anxiety	Decrease in energy	Decreased muscle mass
Delayed healing	Erectile dysfunction	Infertility
Irritability	Loss of interest in sex	Sleeplessness
Small testes	Weight gain	

The Ages and Stages of Manhood

Testosterone pumps strongly in the young 20-year-old male, putting young men in their sexual prime at an early age. Women, on the other hand, do not reach their sexual prime until their late twenties or early thirties.

The chief sex hormone in men is testosterone, produced by the testes, and is important throughout a man's life cycle, including prior to birth. The testes of a male fetus secrete testosterone into the bloodstream. At this time, testosterone influences genital development, as well as the development of the brain and other parts of the body, including the kidneys, the liver, and muscle tissue.

During the first years of life, the young male body does not produce much testosterone, but at puberty, Leydig cells in the testes greatly increase the production of testosterone. At this time, the genitals increase in size, facial hair begins to grow, the voice deepens, muscles increase in size—all changes that mark the transition from childhood to manhood. When less than normal amounts of testosterone are secreted in males, it is said to be a condition known as *testosterone deficiency.*

Balancing the testosterone

Testosterone is the force behind sexual desire and sexual performance. In healthy men, the body produces sufficient testosterone for a lifetime of sexual desire. Testosterone is also responsible for sperm production. In this regard, testosterone is not only important in sexual desire, but also in the ability to reproduce.

But the testes do not continuously pump testosterone into the bloodstream. The hypothalamus and the pituitary gland make gonadotropin-releasing and luteinizing hormones that are necessary to make testosterone. Leydig cells produce testos-

Bright Idea
More than $325 million a year are spent on DHEA and melatonin (natural supplements found at health food stores) to help combat the signs and symptoms of aging. However, it's important to first know the effects and side-effects of such products. Remember, never take a "miracle" cure unless you have thoroughly read the literature and discussed it with your doctor. Most of the time if it sounds too good to be true, it is!

terone, but only when they are stimulated by these other hormones. Like clockwork, responding to levels of testosterone in the bloodstream, the hypothalamus and pituitary gland modify the production of these hormones.

The changes at midlife

During the process of aging, there's a gradual drop in the synthesis of testosterone that may result in numerous physical and mental changes. Whether the signs and symptoms listed in Table 3.3 qualify as "male menopause" is still being debated among scientists. However, if you are a male undergoing any of these changes, you know how they negatively affect your life.

For women, estrogen (female hormone) replacement therapy is now accepted among most physicians and usually has positive results. But the decline in male hormones is usually more gradual and less obvious than the dramatic changes women experience during menopause. This gradual decline makes it difficult to recognize age-related testosterone deficiency. Nonetheless, just as estrogen replacement benefits some post-menopausal women, some researchers are starting to question whether, in some cases, a little testosterone may make a big difference in men.

The replacement debate

Scientists are still debating whether or not testosterone supplements will help aging men. Testosterone revs up the engine of sexual desire and is also responsible for a man's secondary sexual characteristics, including the beard, muscles, thick skin, and possible aggressive attitudes at work.

Testosterone levels might be a key to the effects of aging in men. In fact, any time after age 20 to 30 the level of testosterone begins to decrease in men. It usually continues to gradually decrease, although not a sudden drop as happens with estrogen in women at menopause.

After age 40, low testosterone levels can be common in men. Even though testosterone levels become lower normally, they still may be in the "normal" range. After age 60, in one-third of men, levels of testosterone may drop low enough to cause discernable symptoms, such as a decrease in libido.

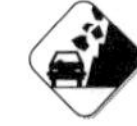

Watch Out!
If your doctor determines that you are deficient in testosterone, make sure that underlying identifiable causes such as testicular problems or pituitary tumors are not present.

The Testosterone–Sex Connection

Along with lower testosterone levels, aging often brings a drop in sexual function, usually experienced as erectile dysfunction. However, aging experts now believe that the drop in testosterone causes loss of desire but not erectile dysfunction in most cases. Your doctor can measure the testosterone level with a blood test. Because of the importance of finding low testosterone levels, men over 50 who have low sexual drive should have their testosterone levels checked. Low testosterone levels can cause other medical problems, such as osteoporosis and loss of muscle strength and mass.

As testosterone levels drop, so does the libido, or sex drive. Fatigue is common, and depression can occur, perhaps as a result of these unwanted changes. When low sex drive and fatigue happen in men, it is worthwhile to check the level of testosterone. The libido can be greatly helped by testosterone treatments. Keep in mind, however, that the problem of erectile dysfunction may be a separate issue that will need to be addressed and treated.

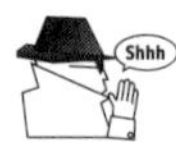

Unofficially... A study of Swedish men found that in men age 50 to 80, 83 percent said sex was very important to them. Although erection problems did increase with age, half of men age 70 to 80 years were still sexually active. One study of American men found that 80 percent age 51 to 64 had sex weekly. And another study of Americans found 80 percent of men over age 69 were still sexually active.

Despite the gradual lowering of testosterone levels even in healthy aging, some men are sexually active into their eighties or even nineties, indicating that there are factors other than testosterone that influence erection and sexual activity.

Less testosterone leads to fewer masculine characteristics

Testosterone is important for maintaining muscles, so as levels of this much-needed male hormone decrease, there may be a drop in muscle size and strength. The drop in testosterone can also lead to hair loss, irritability, forgetfulness, as well as more serious problems such as osteoporosis. Osteoporosis is more common in women, but in fact, 20 to 25 percent of cases occur in men. Osteoporosis in men is linked to low testosterone levels.

Osteoporosis can lead to potentially disabling fractures, but fortunately many of these fractures now can be prevented with proper treatment. After age 75 up to half of men may have osteoporosis, and up to 15 percent of men age 75 to 80 are at risk of hip fracture during their lifetime. Hip fractures from osteoporosis can be devastating, since treatment requires an operation. Up to 50 percent of men with osteoporosis who fall and break a hip after age 75 may die within a year. One-third or more become dependent on others for their daily activities, and many must live in nursing homes.

Gentlemen, know your number

Who doesn't know their blood pressure reading? And, surely you know what your cholesterol level is. But, if you are a male, do you know what your testosterone number is? Especially if you are 40 and above, or if you are experiencing a lack of energy or reduced sex drive, having this level checked by your doctor is important.

When testosterone levels are found to be low, treatment with doses of testosterone can bring levels back to normal, which in turn can increase muscle mass, improve strength, and improve libido. It can also help improve bone mass and prevent or treat osteoporosis. Along with these changes, there is usually an improvement in the overall sense of wellness.

The downside of testosterone supplementation

If testosterone can help this much, why doesn't everyone take it? On one hand, it has been suggested that testosterone supplements can reduce the effects of aging. On the negative side, however, too much testosterone can cause breast development and sterility in men, and even small amounts may contribute to tumor development. Testosterone also increases the production rate of red blood cells, so it could thicken the blood and increase the risk for stroke.

> "When you're impotent, you cannot fake it. My wife can fake arousal, and I'd never know any different. But if I cannot get an erection, nothing I do can make it happen. It's humiliating.
> —Jack, stockbroker, 61"

Another potential side effect of testosterone supplementation is a worsening of prostate enlargement, or possibly even prostate cancer. This could be especially dangerous in patients who have undetected prostate cancer. Researchers recently found that some men with low testosterone levels actually had prostate cancer not detected by the usual rectal exam and PSA test.

In the midst of possible serious side effects, some researchers still say that the benefits are worth the risks because some risks, such as the possibility of heart disease, have not been totally proven.

If your testosterone level proves to be in the low range, then your physician may suggest hormone supplementation. Keep in mind that while some specialists feel that a low testosterone level doesn't necessarily indicate a need for supplementation, others are inclined to try this. Ask your doctor what is best in your situation.

Older Men Can Have Better Sex

The true facts challenge the old myth that sex is out for older Americans. Some researchers have found that although the frequency of sex decreases over time, it was felt to be more enjoyable at an older age, with 75 percent of some groups over age 60 saying that sex was the same or better at that age than when younger.

What's your hurry?

An effect of aging in men is that it may take longer to achieve an erection, which can be used to extend the time of foreplay. This erection may also be less intense. Under these circumstances, it is more important to separate the difference between the physical limits on sex that accompany healthy aging and those resulting from medical problems. Then you can learn to adjust to the age-related sexual problems such as it taking longer to achieve an erection, and at times, less full erections. Because of the drop in sensitivity of the skin of the penis, older men may need longer and more direct stimulation to achieve an erection than in earlier years. Visual stimulation may be less effective, and thoughts that formerly aroused and caused an erection may be slower or less effective. This may be discouraging at first, at least until the man recognizes that it is still possible to achieve an erection. Adjusting to the changes of healthy aging can mean continued satisfying sexual activity.

Close the door on stress

Stress can aggravate less severe problems that might not by themselves create erectile dysfunction. Stress caused by life changes such as divorce or separation, the death of a loved one, changes in work, or problems of children can combine with other factors to result in erectile dysfunction.

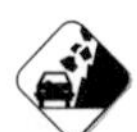

Watch Out!
Believe it or not, some men do experience severe drops in their testosterone levels, resulting in hot flashes and night sweats. It is estimated that between 10 and 15 percent of men have a significant enough drop in testosterone to require hormone replacement therapy.

Move it or lose it

Physical activity often drops after age 50, but it is wrong to assume that exercise, including vigorous exercise, is no longer important. Up to age 80, aging alone has little influence on the overall amount of work and exercise that the heart can do. If no other diseases are present, physical activity and exercise can greatly increase energy, improve overall conditioning, and enhance our capacity for sexual activity.

Sexual activity can also slow down with aging, but as the surveys cited above show, it does not have to decrease. Some studies show that those who have a high level of sexual activity in younger years tend to have a correspondingly high level in later years. Men and women who maintain their level of sexual activity through mid-life tend to keep higher levels of sexual activity in later years.

You Can Run, But You Can't Hide!

The reality of aging cannot be ignored, and there are certain aspects of aging that can affect our sexual function. If we can understand these, make adjustments, and learn to live with the new situation, the reward will be many additional years of active and satisfying sexual activity. If, however, we refuse to accept these facts and maintain the outdated expectations of sexual habits and activities that we had in our twenties, then we may be disappointed that we are unable to stop the tide of physical changes. We may find less sexual satisfaction and more frustration, which can extend to other areas of our lives.

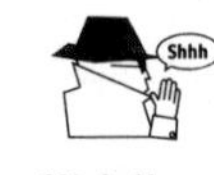

Unofficially... The average potent male has two to five erections during a night's sleep.

Just the Facts

- Many of the most common problems associated with aging can now be slowed or halted with preventative measures.
- As testosterone levels drop with age, fatigue and depression are common symptoms.
- More than $325 million a year are spent on products like DHEA and melatonin to combat signs of aging.
- Some men may benefit from testosterone replacement.
- Thirty percent of the signs of aging are genetically based, but 70 percent are a result of lifestyle habits.

Chapter 4

GET THE SCOOP ON...
The risk factors for heart attack ▪ Impotence as a symptom of coronary artery disease ▪ Heart medicine and erection problems ▪ How exercise and weight loss can fight both heart disease and impotence

The Danger of Heart Disease

Heart disease is the most common cause of serious illness and death in America, with more than 720,000 deaths each year from heart attack due to coronary heart disease. The good news is that if you survive a heart attack, you can gradually return to exercise and daily activities, including sexual activity.

New studies show about half of those who have suffered heart attack return to their previous level of sexual activity. In most cases, the sexual activity was usually begun within eight to 12 weeks after the heart attack.

You may hide your problem with erectile dysfunction from those you love and your doctor, but don't fool around with your ticker as the statistics are serious:

- As many as 1.5 million Americans have heart attacks each year, and about 720,000 of them die.

- More than 15 million Americans are affected by coronary heart disease, and an even larger number don't know that they have heart problems.
- Sixty million people have high blood pressure, a risk factor for heart attack.
- Eighty million people have abnormal cholesterol levels, another important risk factor for heart attack.
- From $50 to $100 billion a year are spent because of heart attack and coronary heart disease.

> "After having a mild heart attack, I made a commitment to stop cigarettes, begin an exercise program for heart patients at the YMCA, and eat for a healthy heart instead of what just tasted good. In six months, I reduced my chances for heart attack immensely. The best news is that the problem I was having with impotence greatly improved once I became physically active again.
> —Zack, building contractor, 54"

While heart attack is the number-one killer in the United States, in many cases, it can be prevented. If you've had a heart attack, it's important to know that living with this affliction does not have to be an ordeal. You can live a normal, productive life, including having an active sex life, by taking measures to reduce the chances of further problems.

What Is Heart Attack?

Heart attack happens when there is a blockage of one of the coronary arteries that supply the heart. When this blockage occurs, the blood and oxygen supply to the heart muscle itself is stopped—and the heart muscle may then stop pumping blood to the brain and other body organs. Or, the heart may begin to have very irregular beats, letting you know that something is off-kilter. These problems are very serious. In fact, each of these problems can cause death if not corrected quickly. If death comes early during a heart attack, the most common cause is the irregular heartbeats.

Unfortunately, death can occur suddenly in coronary heart disease. The most common cause is due to irregular heart beat (arrhythmia), which essentially stops the heart and its pumping action and results in death. There is usually a sudden coronary artery clot and blockage of blood flow.

Researchers have found that 40 to 50 percent of those who have heart attacks may die as a result. Up to 50 percent of those deaths occur in the first few hours, and up to 70 to 80 percent die in the first 24 hours, mainly from the irregular heart beat. While the early hours are most dangerous because of the irregular heart beats, these can be controlled once medical treatment is available. After you are hospitalized, the danger of sudden death decreases because treatment is available.

In many cases, a heart attack is the "last straw" and the "tip of an iceberg." This warning may be the first sign of a heart problem, but it did not just happen. It is one that has been gradually building for years, even though it was invisible and silent. You may have had symptoms or signs, or you may have noticed chest discomfort or shortness of breath when you walk or work.

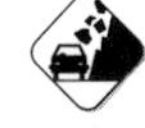

Watch Out!
If you experience intense, unexpected, or prolonged chest pain, call your doctor and get to a hospital emergency room immediately. It may be nothing at all, but why tempt fate?

Heart attacks don't just happen to people at random, but can be linked to specific conditions such as hypertension, high blood cholesterol, or smoking. But heart attacks can be prevented. And you can even predict whether you are at higher risk for a heart attack in the future. This is critical information, since it can also allow you to take steps to prevent heart attack altogether.

First, the arteries narrow

The basic problem in most heart attacks is the narrowing and hardening of the arteries due to atherosclerosis. Again, this process does not happen overnight, but takes years to occur. This narrowing and hardening of the arteries is the same process

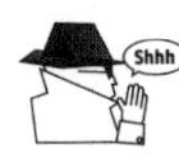

Unofficially... Folic acid found in foods such as spinach is important in preventing heart disease, according to a study in the *Journal of the American Medical Association.*

that can cause heart failure, strokes, and kidney failure. Together these problems are the most common causes of serious illness and death in America. But the leading cause of death is still heart attack.

Researchers think atherosclerosis begins slowly, with minor injuries or wear-and-tear of the inside lining of the arteries, especially the coronary arteries that supply the heart muscle. Changes in flow of blood at branches in the arteries, smoking cigarettes, and high blood cholesterol may all make these minor injuries more likely—and, all of these problems have solutions that only you can control.

FIGURE 4.1: GRADUAL NARROWING AND HARDENING IN A CORONARY ARTERY DUE TO ATHEROSCLEROSIS

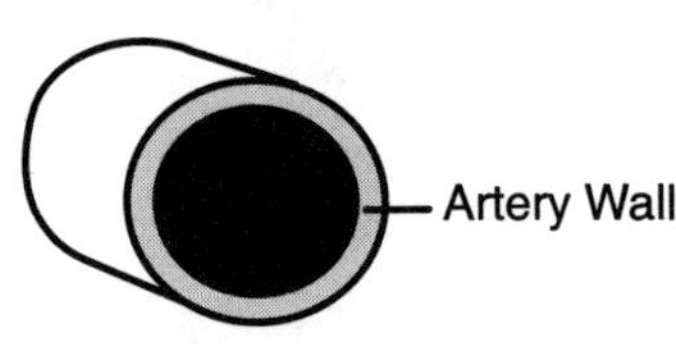

Normal artery with no blockage from atherosclerosis.

At the site of a minor injury there is thought to be a reaction by some of the cells in the blood. This reaction gradually makes the area of injury larger, making it more likely for a clot to form around that area in the blood vessel. Over time, changes from atherosclerosis build up and thicken the wall of the artery. Then, small cracks or fissures form in the same area that further increase the formation of clots, and the arterial narrowing worsens.

A larger clot (thrombosis) can happen suddenly and partially block the flow of blood in the artery. It may even stop blood flow altogether. When this happens there are certain signs and symptoms you may experience.

When the blood flow to the heart muscle is blocked, the heart muscle can become damaged or die, which results in a heart attack (myocardial infarction). The heart beat can become very irregular or the heart muscle may not work normally to pump blood to the body's organs, and heart failure may result.

Who is affected?

More than 15 million Americans are affected by coronary heart disease. Of these 15+ million, more than 1.5 million suffer from heart attack (acute myocardial infarction) each year. One-third of these sufferers, or about 500,000 men and women, die each year from heart attacks. Of the remaining persons who survive heart attack, many are unable to work or have very limited activities.

Watch Out!
Watch your stress load if your blood pressure is elevated. Anxiety, restlessness, tension, tightness, and headaches are all associated with hypertension.

From ages 35 to 44, coronary heart disease is much more common in men than in women—at least six times more common. After menopause, however, heart attacks in women begin to increase. By age 65, women catch up with men in the rate of heart attacks.

As we get older, the risk of death from heart attack also increases. Eighty percent of deaths due to heart attack happen in persons age 65 or older, and most of these actually occur after age 75. Since there are more women than men alive after age 75, the total number of women affected by heart attack during these years is actually greater than the number of men.

Women should be aware that with heart disease, there are times they may be at higher risk than in men. For example, studies have found that the chance of death soon after a heart attack is higher in women than men. And some have found that the chance of death in a hospital is higher in women than in men after coronary bypass surgery. Although no one knows for sure why these statistics are high, some researchers have suggested that more severe coronary blockage or delay in care might account for some of the difference. But it is known that in previous years, the use of certain tests to discover heart disease were less commonly done in women. Talk with your doctor about your individual problems and needs, and make sure that something is being done to diagnose and treat any heart condition.

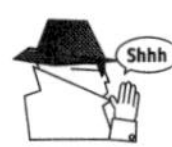

Unofficially... More than 60 million people in the U.S. have blood pressure high enough to raise their risk of heart attack. It has been estimated that at least 10 percent of deaths from coronary heart disease each year could be prevented simply by the treatment of hypertension. This means perhaps 50,000 deaths might be avoided each year.

The overall cost of heart attack is great

The amount of healthcare required increases greatly after a heart attack. Then the cost of health care combined with the loss of work and income places more stress on the patient and family. Estimates are that more than $50 to $100 billion is spent each year on this disease. This cost includes hospitalization, medical treatments, insurance premiums, and loss of work.

Added to this expense is the human cost of suffering in the patient and family. Only those who have experienced heart attack can understand the emotional cost to a loved one who is disabled by this ailment.

Controlling Risk Factors

Certain risk factors can greatly raise one's chances for heart attack. Controlling hypertension, high blood cholesterol, and cigarettes can greatly lower the risk of heart attack, and it is almost never too late in life to take steps to lower risk. For example, control of hypertension and high blood cholesterol have been shown to lower the risk of heart attack up to around age 80. The following is a list of risk factors for heart attack:

- High blood pressure (hypertension)
- High blood cholesterol
- Cigarette smoking
- Diet high in trans-fatty acids
- Lack of exercise
- Being overweight
- Stress (when it is uncontrolled)
- Personality (high levels of hostility and anger)
- Being male
- Age
- Diabetes mellitus
- Family history (i.e., a member who has had a heart attack)

High blood pressure increases your risk

The easiest way to avoid heart attack is to get in control of the risk factors. High blood pressure is a controllable risk factor. If your blood pressure remains above the normal level, you should take steps to control it. For instance, eating a low-salt diet and getting exercise can treat hypertension without medication, although in many cases, medication may also be needed.

Watch Out!
Remember that some medications for hypertension also have impotence as a side effect. Let your doctor guide you for the medication that is best for your situation.

According to a USDA survey, the average American consumes a whopping 6,600 mg of sodium each day. That is only one tablespoon of salt, but it is two and a half times the recommended daily maximum of 2,400 mg. The facts about sodium and the American way of life are startling:

- Many persons with hypertension could lower their blood pressure by limiting sodium.
- 80 percent of Americans' sodium intake comes from processed foods.

Inasmuch as people consume more than the daily maximum of salt, the body's needs are subsequently less. The actual needs are only about $^{1}/_{2}$ to 1 teaspoon of salt per day (1,100 to 3,300 mg sodium). For the 50 to 60 million Americans with high blood pressure, reducing the amount of salt in the diet could help some people avoid this ailment.

TABLE 4.1: CATEGORIES OF HYPERTENSION

Systolic (upper number)	**Diastolic (lower number)**	
Normal Blood Pressure	less than 130	less than 85
High normal	130-139	85-89
Hypertension		
Stage 1 (mild)	140-159	90-99
Stage 2 (moderate)	160-179	100-109
Stage 3 (severe)	180-209	110-119
Stage 4 (very severe)	210 or higher	120 or higher

Although the words "salt" and "sodium" are often used interchangeably, they are not the same. Ordinary table salt is only 40 percent sodium. Too much sodium can increase fluid retention and elevate blood pressure in people who are sodium sensitive.

Many foods naturally contain sodium, including animal products like meat, fish, poultry, milk, and eggs. Vegetable products are naturally low in sodium. Most of the sodium in our diets, however, comes from commercially processed foods such as cured meats like bacon and ham, luncheon meats, sausage, frozen breaded meats, fish and seafood, and canned meats. Condiments like catsup, mustard, and steak sauce are also high in sodium. Fast foods such as hamburgers, french fries, and prepare-at-home fast foods like frozen pizza, hot dogs, sausage, creamed chipped beef, and broccoli with cheese sauce are very high in sodium. Start reading the nutritional label on the package to determine the sodium content, and make it a point to stay within recommended limits.

Bright Idea
Eating a lot of high-potassium foods such as orange juice, potatoes, and bananas may help to reduce high blood pressure, a risk factor for heart attack.

Words that have soda, sodium, or "Na" associated with them indicate sodium as a part of a preservative or flavoring agent. Some examples are monosodium glutamate, baking soda, sodium nitrate, sodium propionate, and sodium benzoate.

The U.S. Food and Drug Administration (FDA) requires nutrient labels on food packages to list the sodium content. Terms such as "low sodium" and "sodium free" are also standardized to help the conscientious consumer. See Table 4.2.

TABLE 4.2: FDA STANDARDIZED SODIUM LABEL REQUIREMENTS

Sodium free	Less than 5 mg sodium/serving
Very low sodium	35 mg or less sodium/serving
Low sodium	140 mg or less sodium/serving
Reduced sodium	Sodium reduced 75% compared to the product it is replacing
Unsalted	No salt added. Sodium has not been used in processing

Sodium is measured in grams and milligrams (mg). A gram is a unit of weight. There are about 28 grams in one ounce. One gram equals 1,000 milligrams. Try not to exceed 2,000 milligrams a day, or talk to your doctor about personal limitations of sodium. (See Table 4.3 for a list of high-sodium foods to avoid.)

Other ways to reduce your risk for heart attack include:

- Control your weight to control your blood pressure. Even losing five to ten pounds can significantly reduce blood pressure (see Chapter 16).
- Begin a regular exercise program to lower blood pressure.
- Manage stress to lower blood pressure.
- Reduce excess alcohol intake to lower blood pressure.
- Maintain an adequate intake of potassium and calcium to lower blood pressure (see Tables 4.4 and 4.5 for a list of foods high in potassium and calcium). The recommended calcium intake for adult men 25-64 years old is 1,000 milligrams per day. This increases to 1,500 milligrams per day after age 65. Taking more than is recommended could be harmful, so talk with your doctor.

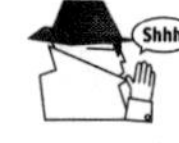

Unofficially... Heart Disease is the number one killer in the United States and often has no symptoms.

If you cannot reduce your blood pressure using these natural methods, then talk with your doctor about a medication that would help you—without the side effect of impotence.

TABLE 4.3: SODIUM CONTENT OF SELECTED FOODS

Food	Amount	Milligrams
Bacon	2 slices	200
Baking powder	1 tsp.	339
Baking soda	1 tsp.	821
Beans, green	1/2 cup	230
Beef broth	1 cube	1,150
Beef, lean	3 ounces cooked	55
Bread	1 slice	150
Biscuit	1 (2" diameter)	220
Buttermilk	1 cup	330
Cereal, dry, flake	2/3 cup	200
Cheeseburger, fast food	1/4 lb.	1,200
Chicken noodle soup	1 cup	1,100
Cornbread	1 small square	260
Cheese, American	1 ounce	400
Cheese, cheddar	1 ounce	200
Cheese, mozzarella, part-skim	1 ounce	132
Chocolate shake	1 average	300
Cottage cheese	4 ounces	450
Frankfurter	1	500
Garlic powder	1 tsp.	1
Garlic salt	1 tsp.	1,850
Ham	3 ounces	1,000
Ketchup	1 tbl.	156
Lite salt	1/4 tsp.	250
Luncheon meat	1 slice	575
Mayonnaise	1 tbl.	80
Meat tenderizer	1 tsp.	1,750
MSG, flavor enhancer	1/4 tsp.	50
Mustard	1 tsp.	65
Oatmeal, instant	3/4 cup	240
Oatmeal, regular	3/4 cup	1
Olives, green	3	720
Onion powder	1 tsp.	1
Onion salt	1 tsp.	1,620
Peas, green canned	1 cup	493
Peas, green frozen	1 cup	150
Potato, boiled	1 cup	7

Table Continues

Timesaver
If you don't have time to add fish to your meals, take fish oil capsules, which are high in omega-3 fatty acids. These are available at most grocery and drug stores. Ask your doctor for the recommended dosage.

Bright Idea
You can prevent heart disease by eliminating known risk factors by quitting cigarettes; reducing cholesterol, triglycerides, and blood pressure to normal limits; losing weight; and increasing exercise.

Food	Amount	Milligrams
Potato, instant	1 cup	475
Potato chips	1 ounce	300
Peanut butter	1 tbl.	100
Sauerkraut	2/3 cup	740
Sausage, pork	2 links	380
Salt	1/4 tsp.	500
Soy sauce	1 tbsp.	1,030
Tomato juice	1 cup	210

While you are calculating your salt intake, there are also certain foods to avoid, including:

- Canned and dried soups
- Canned vegetables
- Canned meats (tuna, chicken, etc.)
- Ketchup, mustard, barbecue, steak, and soy sauces
- Salty snack foods (potato chips, nuts, etc.)
- Luncheon meats and packaged foods
- Olives and pickles
- Bacon, cured meats, ham
- Cheese and cheese products
- Fast foods (french fries, onion rings, hamburgers, Chinese food)

TABLE 4.4: FOODS HIGH IN POTASSIUM

Apricots (fresh, dried)	Avocados	Bananas	Buttermilk
Cantaloupe	Chicken	Cod	Great Northern beans (cooked)
Flounder	Milk (skim, whole)	Orange juice	Peaches
Potatoes	Raisins	Salmon (fresh, cooked)	Sardines
Sweet potatoes	Tomatoes (raw)	Turkey	

TABLE 4.5: COMMON FOODS WITH HIGH CALCIUM CONTENT

Food	Amount	Calcium content
Beans, baked	1 cup	150
Beans, black	1 cup	250
Broccoli	1 cup	145
Cabbage, steamed	1 cup	65
Cheese, cheddar	1 cup	845
Cheese, Monterey jack	1 ounce	200
Cheese, reduced calorie, low-fat	1 ounce	200
Cottage cheese	1 cup	140
Chocolate milk (1% milk fat)	8 ounces	300
Evaporated condensed milk	8 ounces	800
Evaporated skim milk	8 ounces	500-600
Ice cream	1 cup	175-270
Kale	1 cup	205
Milk, cow's milk	8 ounces	500
Milk, cow's, skim	8 ounces	300
Okra, steamed	1 cup	150
Spinach, steamed	1 cup	170
Sweet potato, canned	1 cup	85
Turnip greens	1 cup	270
Yogurt	8 ounces	300
Frozen yogurt	6 ounces	150

Abnormal blood cholesterol also increases risk

Cholesterol is normally present in the blood. When the body produces too much, or when the levels are too high from other causes, the risk of coronary heart disease increases accordingly. This is because high cholesterol levels contribute to the development of atherosclerosis—especially in the coronary arteries (see Figure 4.2).

FIGURE 4.2: THE RISK OF HEART ATTACK AS THE FUNCTION OF TOTAL CHOLESTEROL

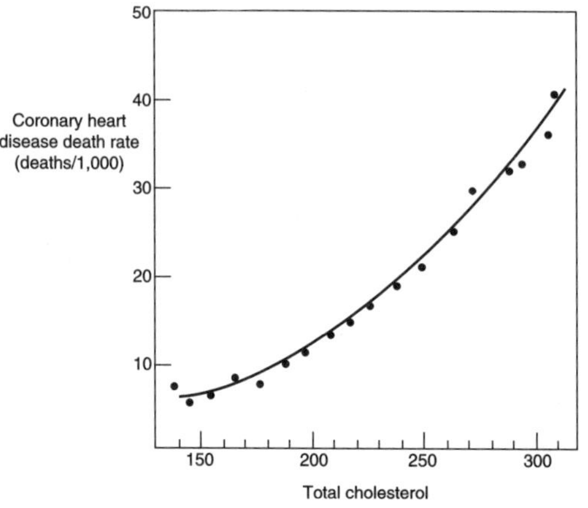

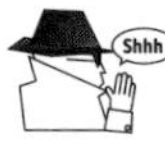

Unofficially... The new DASH (Dietary Approaches to Stop Hypertension) diet has been found to reduce blood pressure in about two weeks. The daily diet includes seven to eight servings of grain or grain products, four to five servings of fruit, four to five servings of vegetables, two to three servings of nonfat or low-fat dairy products, 1/2 serving of nuts, and two or fewer servings of lean meat.

Normal total cholesterol is that below 200 mg/dl. However, up to one-half of those who have already had a heart attack, coronary artery bypass, or angioplasty may have cholesterol levels in this "normal" range, while their other types of cholesterol went unmeasured.

The risk of heart attack increases gradually as the total cholesterol level increases above 200. Fifty to 80 percent of men in some studies have cholesterol levels higher than this. Testing for high-density lipoprotein (HDL) cholesterol and low-density lipoprotein (LDL) cholesterol is also needed.

About 80 million Americans have high blood cholesterol, which also increases the risk of heart attack. For example, the risk of heart attack has been found to increase when cholesterol levels are above 200 mg/dl. The risk doubles if the cholesterol level is above 240–265 (see Figure 4.2). Actually, most heart attacks happen with the total cholesterol level between 200 and 240 ("borderline high"), and about 15 percent of heart attacks happen in people whose total cholesterol is below 200, or "normal."

High blood cholesterol may be successfully treated with a low-cholesterol diet. If diet alone does not control high blood cholesterol, then your doctor can help decide whether you should take medication to lower cholesterol. Studies show that controlling high blood cholesterol up to age 80 is effective in lowering the risk of heart attack.

Bright Idea
If you have high cholesterol, keep in mind that you are what you eat! A diet high in saturated fat (found in meat and dairy products) and transfatty acids (found in margarine, snack and fast foods, crackers, pastries, and many processed foods) can lead to heart disease, as well as obesity and some types of cancer.

TABLE 4.6: KNOW YOUR NUMBER

Total Cholesterol	
Desirable	less than 200*
Borderline high	200-239
High	240 or higher
*(this may vary and still be desirable, depending on HDL cholesterol and LDL cholesterol)	
LDL Cholesterol	
Desirable (for person with coronary heart disease)	100 or less
Desirable	130 or less
Borderline high	130-159
High	160 or higher
HDL Cholesterol	
Desirable to lower risk	60 or higher
Persons at higher heart risk	less than 35

Watch your dietary cholesterol

Your cholesterol level can be directly affected by cholesterol in the diet. By lowering your blood cholesterol level, you dramatically reduce your risk of coronary heart disease.

Dietary cholesterol is found in animal foods—meats, poultry, fish, egg yolks, milk, cream, cheese, butter, and other dairy foods.

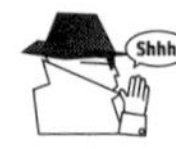

Unofficially... If you are worried about having sex after a heart attack, talk to your doctor. New research has shown that sex stresses the heart less than walking up two flights of stairs or merging into freeway traffic during rush hour, especially if the lover with heart disease is on the bottom. Heart attacks are very rare during and shortly after sex.

Smoking: a risk factor you can change

Smoking cigarettes increases the risk of heart attack, as well as other health problems (see Table 4.8). However, there is a quick drop in risk after quitting. While it may be hard to quit, there are many innovative ways to break this habit, including individual and group counseling, medications including nicotine patches, and other methods that can be successful. Talk to your physician for advice.

Other risk factors for heart attack are listed above. It would be a good idea to check your risk factors annually, then ask your doctor for advice on how to control each one. This is a chance to prevent more complicated, limiting and expensive medical problems and to improve your quality of life.

The health risks caused by smoking are:

- Coronary heart disease, especially heart attack and heart failure.
- Magnifies the risk for coronary heart disease in those who already have high risk from hypertension and high blood cholesterol.
- Atherosclerosis and blockage of the arteries that supply the feet and legs—leading to gangrene and amputation.
- Atherosclerosis and blockage of the arteries that supply blood to the brain—leading to stroke.
- Increased risk of sudden death.
- Blood cholesterol increased by increasing the LDL-cholesterol and may decrease the HDL-cholesterol.
- Decreased physical performance, endurance, and lung function.

TABLE 4.7: CHOLESTEROL CONTENT OF SELECTED FOODS

Food	Amount	Milligrams
Dairy		
Butter	1 tsp.	11
Cheese, American	1 ounce	16
Cheese, mozzarella, part skim	1 ounce	15
Cottage cheese, 1% fat	1 cup	10
Cream	1 tbl.	20
Milk, 1%	1 cup	10
Milk, skim	1 cup	5
Sherbet	1/2 cup	7
Margarine	1 tsp.	0
Cheese, cheddar	1 ounce	30
Cheese, Swiss	1 ounce	26
Half-and-half	1 tbl.	6
Milk, 2%	1 cup	18
Milk, whole	1 cup	34
Ice cream	1/2 cup	30
Poultry		
Chicken, dark (no skin)	3 ounces	81
Turkey, dark (no skin)	3 ounces	87
Chicken, white (no skin)	3 ounces	72
Turkey, white (no skin)	3 ounces	66
Red meat		
Bacon	1 slice	5
Frankfurter	1.6 ounces	45
Pork (lean)	3 ounces	75

Table continues

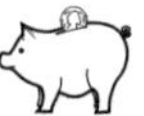

Moneysaver
If you are taking fish oil capsules for heart health, try eating more fish with your meals to save money. Studies show that fish such as mackerel, bluefish, tuna, herring, anchovies, sardines or salmon are high in omega-3 fatty acids, which have been shown to reduce the "bad" LDL-cholesterol and raise the "good" HDL-cholesterol.

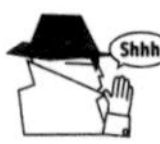

Unofficially... Heart attacks have a 50 percent death rate if they happen outside of the hospital, usually from very irregular heart beats, which can be treated if discovered.

Food	Amount	Milligrams
Red meat		
Beef, lean	3 ounces	78
Ham (boiled)	3 ounces	75
Veal (lean)	3 ounces	84
Seafood/fish		
Crab	3 ounces	85
Haddock	3 ounces	40
Oysters	3 ounces	42
Tuna	3 ounces	55
Flounder	3 ounces	70
Lobster	3 ounces	70
Shrimp	3 ounces	128
Breads/Cereals/Grains		
Bread	1 slice	0
Doughnut, raised	1	21
Rice, plain	$^1/_2$ cup	0
Bagel	1 whole	0
Oatmeal	$^1/_2$ cup	0
Cookie, plain	1	1
Fruits/Vegetables		
Potato, baked	1 small	0
Cabbage	$^1/_2$ cup	0
Banana	1 medium	0
Potato, fried	10 fries	0
Apple	1 medium	0

What You May Feel

Most of us are familiar with the commonly known symptoms of heart attack—severe pain in the chest, numbing of the left arm, shortness of breath. Nonetheless, did you know that you can have a heart attack without any unusual feelings at all? Do you know when to call a doctor when you do have an unusual symptom, one that might be related to your heart? And do you know which symptoms must be treated so there will be no further danger to your heart health?

It is important to understand all of the warning signs of coronary heart disease or heart attack. If treated in the earliest stages, you increase your chances for survival without permanent damage and for living a normal, active life.

Remember that the more risk factors you have, the higher the chances are that you might develop coronary heart disease. Being aware of risk factors is important to your long-term health. Early detection is also important if you develop heart disease, since many of the complications can be prevented.

The most common first sign of coronary heart disease is discomfort in the chest. This can be a sensation of tightness, pressure, dull pain, squeezing, heaviness, aching, indigestion, burning or other discomfort, or a combination of any of these. It can happen at rest or may only happen with some exertion such as walking, working, lifting, or after a large meal. This might even come on when you are not active, especially at night, and it may awaken you from sleep. Some notice these feelings first during sudden change in activity such as shoveling snow after the first snowstorm.

The chest pain or discomfort may move around and might be felt in a shoulder, arm, neck, jaw, or back. At times, there may only be discomfort in the shoulder or arm, with little or no pain in the chest. There may be shortness of breath, which is usually mild. This usually disappears along with the chest discomfort. Some persons also have sweating or nausea. This might come on when you are not active, especially at first, or the sweating and nausea might awaken you from sleep.

Do not ignore symptoms

In some cases it will be easy to overlook or ignore the feelings. You may have only arm or jaw pain, or the feeling might be ignored as only indigestion.

When any of the chest discomfort above is caused by coronary heart disease it is called *angina pectoris*. The feelings usually last only a few minutes. Sitting and resting for a few minutes or taking nitroglycerin medication may provide relief. At times the activity that causes the pain can be predicted and avoided. For instance, some persons find that it only comes on if they are walking too fast, walking uphill, or walking in cold weather. Some only notice it if they do all three—walk too fast, uphill, and in cold weather!

TABLE 4.8: COMMON SYMPTOMS OF HEART ATTACK

A feeling in the chest of			
Tightness	Pressure	Dull pain	Squeezing
Heaviness	Aching	Indigestion	Burning
Or other discomfort or a combination of any of these.			
Pain felt in the			
Shoulders	Arms	Neck	Jaw
Back			
Also			
Shortness of breath			
Nausea and sweating			

Call your doctor

Any of the signs listed in Table 4.8 should alert you to talk to your doctor. If it is the first time for the feeling or if it lasts for more than a few minutes, then call immediately. If you know you have coronary heart disease, and the discomfort lasts longer than usual or comes on more often than usual, you should call your doctor or immediately dial 911.

Don't ignore or deny these feelings—check them out with your doctor. Don't be embarrassed to tell what may seem like trivial or meaningless signs or feelings. These may be the only warning signs of serious coronary heart disease you ever have!

Even if you have none of the risk factors discussed above, do not hesitate to call your doctor if you have chest discomfort. It is too important to miss this problem early when treatment is best. If there is any question, or you are not sure what to do, call your doctor or go to an emergency room for evaluation.

Don't ever be too embarrassed about seeking treatment. The earlier you seek care, the better the treatment is likely to be. Excellent treatment is available, once the diagnosis is made.

Watch Out!
There may be no feeling of chest pain or discomfort at all with "silent" ischemia. It is very common and just as serious as when there is chest discomfort. Silent ischemia is detected by special testing, so talk to your doctor if there is concern, especially if you are diabetic.

Types of angina pectoris

There are several types of angina pectoris. Stable angina pectoris means that the discomfort and limitation have not increased recently, such as over the previous one to two months. There may be chest pain, tightness, or other discomfort on exertion or from other causes, but the severity and frequency of the episodes are the same. The chest discomfort usually lasts less than five minutes and is relieved by resting or by nitroglycerin medication.

> "I had chest pains the last two times I was playing golf. I honestly thought they would go away and ignored them, but at the time of my routine check-up, I decided I better talk about it with my doctor. After doing tests, my doctor said I had blockage of a major degree in one coronary artery, with the others showing little change. I had successful angioplasty with a balloon tipped catheter and have now returned to golf without any limitations.
> —Simon, professor, 59"

In persons with stable angina, researchers usually find a narrowing of at least one of the coronary arteries. The narrowed blood vessel allows enough blood (and oxygen) to reach the heart muscle when at rest. With more activities, however, the heart increases its work and needs more blood, but the narrowed vessel limits the supply of blood, and angina develops. With rest, the need for more blood lessens, and the chest pain goes away. Medication such as nitroglycerin may relieve the pain in a few minutes, and other medications can help prevent angina. Your doctor needs to guide your treatment.

Angina pectoris is called "unstable" when the chest discomfort changes—if it happens for the first time or when it becomes more frequent or longer lasting. Being aware of this change is important because it means danger with a higher risk of sudden worsening of the coronary heart disease at this time.

In unstable angina pectoris, the chest discomfort may happen more often or with much less activity or less exertion than usual. It commonly happens with no activity at all—even simply awakening from sleep. Unstable angina pectoris can happen after a heart attack or in a patient who has already had coronary heart disease, such as coronary artery surgery.

Unstable angina pectoris can happen suddenly with no specific cause, even when you have done everything as prescribed. Patients need immediate medical attention and hospitalization during any of the above types of unstable angina pectoris or prolonged chest pain.

Researchers have found that in unstable angina pectoris there is usually a sudden decrease in the blood flow in a coronary artery. This can happen from a small crack or fissure in the wall of the artery. The fissure causes a reaction nearby, which results in a clot in the artery with temporary blockage of the blood flow. The actual event that causes the crack or fissure is not known.

Prolonged chest pain

If the chest discomfort lasts longer than 20 minutes, then it is also treated as unstable angina pectoris, especially in a person who has had a heart attack or coronary artery surgery in the past. At this time, there is a higher risk of sudden death from heart attack due to irregular heart beat.

Unstable angina can lead to heart attack

Any of the types of unstable angina pectoris discussed above can lead to heart attack. Fortunately, most of the time unstable angina does not lead to actual death of heart muscle. However, if the blood flow continues to be severely limited or stopped altogether for a long enough time, then there may be actual death of some of the heart muscle and myocardial infarction.

Heart attack can also happen with no earlier warning signs at all. In up to one-third of heart attacks, unstable angina is the first sign of coronary disease. The chest discomfort may be sudden, severe, and dramatic. Some describe feeling as if "an elephant is sitting on my chest." Others tell of having the feeling of a "hot poker" through the chest. Still others have only mild tightness, pressure, or indigestion. Any of the feelings described above for angina pectoris can happen in heart attack.

The discomfort usually lasts more than a few minutes but may last for hours. It is dangerous to wait at home when these feelings occur. This is the period of highest risk in heart attack.

The chest discomfort may travel to one or both arms or to the neck or jaw. At times, there may be only pain in an arm or jaw with no noticeable chest pain. Dizziness may be present and the patient may collapse, especially if the heart rhythm is irregular.

There is often shortness of breath with a feeling of suffocation. Sweating is common and may even be the first sign. There may be nausea, vomiting, or a feeling of the need to have a bowel movement.

Unofficially... The FDA warns that it is dangerous to take the impotence pill Viagra together with nitroglycerin or related heart drugs. If you take any heart medication, discuss this with your doctor before trying Viagra.

Most critical in the successful treatment of heart attack is timing. Since the first one to two hours are the time when most deaths occur due to heart attack, it is extremely important to get medical attention quickly. Call 911 or your local emergency medical service. This is the time when it is very common for a patient to delay getting proper care. The reasons range from denying there is a problem to not wanting to be trouble to anyone. Many times a family member or friend helps make the decision to get emergency care.

Making the Diagnosis of Heart Attack

Your doctor will make the diagnosis of heart attack (myocardial infarction) after taking your medical history, doing a full physical examination, and doing an electrocardiogram (ECG or EKG), as well as other specific tests.

There may be permanent ECG changes (called Q-wave infarction) that indicate a more complete and longer-lasting blockage of the coronary artery and possibly death of heart muscle. In most cases, this is thought to be due to a larger crack or fissure in the wall of the artery, which causes a more severe clot.

In myocardial infarction there may be no permanent ECG changes (called non-Q-wave infarction). Researchers believe that this is because the blockage of the blood vessel did not last long enough, or because other arteries made up for the loss of blood supply. In this type of myocardial infarction, there may be less actual permanent damage or death in the heart muscle itself. However, there is still risk in the future.

Impotence as a Sign of Heart Disease

Men who develop impotence because of blood flow problems may have underlying heart disease even though they are not experiencing any other symptoms, according to some researchers. As discussed, impotence may also be the first sign of diabetes. It can also be a sign of kidney failure, or neurological diseases such as multiple sclerosis and lumbar disc disorders.

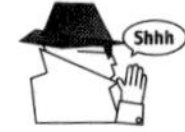

Unofficially...

Heart attacks can happen at any time of day or night, but are most common in morning hours, around 5 a.m. until noon. This happens to be when the blood pressure is also commonly higher.

New findings that link impotence and heart disease provide another important reason why men should undergo a thorough health examination rather than simply take measures or medications like Viagra to treat the impotency.

Some researchers found that almost 40 percent of men had erectile dysfunction after a heart attack. Anxiety and depression (see Chapter 10) are thought to play a role in erection problems after heart attack, although medications used to treat heart disease may also contribute to erection problems, including medications for hypertension. Sources of anxiety are the fear of performance failure in the sexual activity and fear of another heart attack or even death during sex.

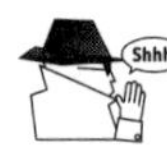

Unofficially... In a study of 42 middle-aged men, researchers found that those patients whose impotence was associated with a problem of penile blood flow were more likely to have an abnormality discovered by a cardiologist during a stress test even though they reported no symptoms other than the impotence.

Some patients are limited in physical activity after a heart attack, which may in turn limit sexual performance. The exertion involved in sexual activity may be enough to cause heart attack in less than one in 100 cases, and the risk of death during sex is probably one or two in one million. The bottom line is that the overall risk of heart attack during sex is low—but you should openly discuss this with your doctor to evaluate your overall situation.

Medications that are necessary for the heart disease may also contribute to erection problems. Diuretics commonly prescribed for heart failure due to coronary heart disease may add to erection difficulty.

The medication Viagra can be dangerous in patients with coronary heart disease and other forms of heart disease.

Factors in the high rate of impotence

Researchers have found that loss of interest and desire, the lack of spouse's cooperation, depression, and fear of a return of the heart disease or death were also factors in slowing a return to sexual activity. Similar problems happen after a heart attack, after angioplasty, and after coronary artery bypass graft surgery. After coronary artery bypass grafting there is also soreness in the chest, which lasts eight weeks or more.

Treating erectile dysfunction in heart patients

Treatment of erectile dysfunction when it is linked to coronary heart disease starts with controlling the heart problem and taking the important steps to lower your risk of future heart attack. Your family physician and cardiologist can stabilize your condition and guide the cardiac rehabilitation program.

As your exercise and rehabilitation progress, your doctor can tell you when it's safe for sexual activity. If you have erection problems, consider eliminating any risk factors you can control (cigarette smoking, alcohol use, certain medications, and stress).

It's important that you talk to your doctor, decide the most likely cause of the problem, and begin treatment if it continues. If your doctor is not comfortable discussing your erection problem, he or she can help you find a person who can advise you. Researchers and counselors have found that it is best when patients are reassured that their thoughts, feelings, and desires about returning to sexual activity are normal.

Watch Out!
Those who take nitroglycerin or nitrate-related medications SHOULD NOT TAKE VIAGRA. The combination of medication can cause dramatic drops in blood pressure and in some patients, the drop may be critical for the heart or brain. This may result in heart attack, stroke, and even death.

It is good to ask questions and get information about your own situation. This will increase the chances that your return to full activity after coronary heart disease includes a return to a satisfying sexual life, as well. Specific recommendations for your own situation might include timing of sexual activity (morning or evening), avoiding sex when fatigued, or when under emotional stress. Some positions cause less work on the heart than others and may be helpful in preventing recurrence of chest pain or shortness of breath.

Knowing which warning signs to report to your doctor is important, such as chest pain or shortness of breath during or after sexual activity. Having the facts can give peace of mind, lower anxiety

Heart Disease Is Treatable

Heart disease, especially coronary heart disease, can be treated and steps can be taken to prevent future heart attacks. A guided program of exercise and rehabilitation can restore your usual daily activities including sexual activities. Treatment is available for erectile dysfunction, but be certain that you are not taking any medications that might conflict with impotence drugs, such as Viagra.

Again, as in all chronic illnesses and their link with impotence, the main ingredient in the treatment and prevention is you. In other words, you can change things in your life so that the chances of having sexual problems are greatly reduced.

Just the Facts

- Fifteen million Americans suffer from coronary artery disease. Of this 15 million, more than 1.5 million suffer from heart attack (acute myocardial infarction) each year. One-third of these sufferers, about 500,000 men and women, die each year from heart attacks.

- Heart disease costs more than $50 to $100 billion each year due to hospitalization, medical treatments, insurance premiums, and loss of work.

- Some natural ways to reduce blood pressure include staying at a normal weight, increasing exercise, staying on a low-salt diet, increasing calcium and potassium, and watching excess stress.

- Men who develop impotence because of blood flow problems may have underlying heart disease even though they are not experiencing any other symptoms.

- Research shows that more than 40 percent of men have erectile dysfunction after suffering heart attack.

Chapter 5

GET THE SCOOP ON...

How diabetes can go undetected until severe enough to require hospitalization ▪ How to control diabetes-related complications, including those that lead to erectile dysfunction ▪ How 75 percent of new cases of type 2 diabetes can be prevented ▪ How Viagra may benefit diabetics who are impotent because of nerve damage to the penis

The Menace of Diabetes

Many chronic diseases associated with aging sneak up on you with no warning signs until it is too late. Take diabetes, for example.

More than 20 million Americans may have this very serious disease, yet many do not know they are affected because they have not yet had symptoms. In most cases, there are no obvious feelings or signs until the blood glucose gradually increases to become high enough to cause fatigue, increased thirst and urination, blurred vision, weight loss, and eventually serious illness, which may be severe enough to need hospitalization.

According to the Centers for Disease Control and Prevention, the prevalence of diabetes is rising as the U.S. population ages and as more Americans become obese. While the actual cause of diabetes is not known, excellent treatment that can control the symptoms is available. As we have already discussed, the best way to prevent complications with any chronic illness is to take charge—get an accurate diagnosis, treat the symptoms early when they are most likely to respond, and manage the disease just as you manage other parts of your life.

The problem with diabetes is the myriad complications you will experience if treatment is delayed. For example, you may have kidney damage, a higher risk of atherosclerosis with coronary heart disease, and blockage of the arteries to the legs, damage to the nerves, especially those that supply the legs and feet. Impotence affects more than 50 to 60 percent of all men with this disease.

Early Detection Is the Key

Early detection to allow treatment and prevention of complications is so important that the American Diabetes Association recently recommended that all persons over age 45 have a blood glucose test every three years.

A simple blood test for glucose can tell if you are diabetic. The diagnosis of diabetes is made when the blood glucose is 126 mg/dl or greater on two separate testing occasions after not eating overnight. Or, if the blood glucose is 200 mg/dl or more two hours after a standard meal, then diabetes is present.

Take diabetes seriously

If your doctor tells you that you have diabetes or are a "borderline" diabetic, take it seriously. You can control the complications, including those that lead to erectile dysfunction, if you control your weight, exercise regularly, eat a reasonable diet, and, if needed, take the medication to control blood glucose. The goal is to try to keep the blood glucose controlled at 140 mg/dl or less.

With diabetes, it is the long-term complications that cause damage to internal organs. These include the following:

- Kidney disease
- Blindness
- Nerve damage
- A higher risk of atherosclerosis in blood vessels of the heart, kidney, legs, brain, and other organs
- There can also be damage to nerves, including the nerves that supply internal organs, pelvic organs, and those that allow erections

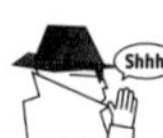

Unofficially... Diabetics have up to four times the chance of death from coronary heart disease. About half of the foot and leg amputations not related to injury occur in diabetics, and diabetic kidney disease is the leading cause of renal failure in the United States.

Diabetes contributes to more than 250,000 deaths a year. More than 90 percent of people with the disease have type 2 diabetes. The main risk factor for type 2 diabetes is obesity, and a prime cause of obesity is a high-fat diet.

The nation's leading cause of death—heart disease—kills 720,000 Americans a year, most as a result of heart attacks. Compared with non-diabetics, people with diabetes have three times the risk of heart disease. A high-fat diet is a key cause of the cholesterol-rich deposits called plaques that narrow the coronary arteries and trigger heart attacks. Virtually all Americans, especially diabetics, have these plaques in their coronary arteries. These plaques begin to develop as soon as people start eating a high-fat diet, which in America means during childhood.

Obesity leads to type 2 diabetes

"Obese" means weighing 20 percent more than the recommended weight for your height and build. Obesity is the prime risk factor for type 2 diabetes.

It also increases risk of heart disease, several cancers, hypertension, and arthritis. It is a problem only in countries with a high-fat diet.

The most common type of diabetes, type 2, does not require insulin for treatment. It is most common after age 55. Most diabetics with type 2 diabetes have one risk factor in common—they are overweight.

Bright Idea
For all those with type 2 diabetes, treatment includes proper diet and exercise to control weight and blood glucose. Your doctor can guide you to excellent blood glucose control, which means keeping the blood glucose as close as possible to normal most of the time.

Obesity greatly increases the risk for diabetes, as does having an affected family member. African-Americans are also at higher risk. In fact, African-Americans are twice as likely to have diabetes as the general population, and the rate of diagnosed diabetes in the African-American community has tripled in the past 30 years, according to the American Diabetes Association.

The exact cause of diabetes is not known, but some of the factors are thought to be changes in the body's metabolism with age, made worse by being overweight and by not exercising.

Fifteen percent of diabetics have type 1

The other major type of diabetes, type 1 diabetes, requires insulin to control blood glucose. Fifteen percent of the 16 to 20 million Americans with diabetes have this type of diabetes. About 15 percent of diabetics are type 1. It has been shown that good control of blood glucose lowers the risk for complications such as nerve damage, kidney disease, and heart disease. This type of diabetes also puts you at high risk for nerve damage, including the nerves which supply the penis and allow erection.

The good and bad news

Not only is diabetes the fourth leading cause of death in the U.S., it kills more people each year than either AIDS or breast cancer. Studies show that if you are diagnosed with diabetes in your forties or fifties, it could shorten your life by as much as five to ten years. You could also become blind or lose kidney function and have to be put on a dialysis machine. The good news is that more than 75 percent of the new cases of type 2 diabetes can be prevented.

Diabetes and Erectile Dysfunction

Fifty to 60 percent of diabetic men over age 50 have erectile dysfunction at some time. Erection problems may even be the first sign of diabetes. It is thought that the continuous high blood glucose level affects the nerves that supply the penis and allow erection. This is usually a temporary problem and when the blood glucose becomes normal or closer to normal, erections can resume as before. If the blood glucose is controlled by following the proper diet and taking prescribed medications, there may no more problems with erection.

Case study of typical middle-aged diabetic

David is 52 years old and had not had a physical examination for over 10 years. He had finally agreed to have the exam after six months of increasing tiredness. David felt tired when he awoke in the morning, and it became worse during the day. Shortly before his exam, he had noticed blurred vision and planned to have his eyes checked to see if his glasses needed to be changed.

David became concerned about his health after he had difficulty maintaining an erection. This was a problem he had never experienced, even though he felt the desire for sex as much as ever. Over the previous two months he also noticed that he urinated more frequently than usual.

The physical exam revealed no problems except for his weight of 240 pounds (height 5'8"). His blood pressure was normal, and all of his other blood tests were normal except the blood glucose, which was 325 mg/dl. He had never been diabetic, but he had a sister who had been diagnosed with diabetes a few years earlier. He had not had a blood test in 10 years.

With a goal of gradual weight loss, David began a diet that he found easy to live with. He began a walking program and took medication to control the blood glucose. He started checking his own blood glucose at home and found that with the diet, weight loss, and medication, his blood glucose dropped to normal levels in about three months. During this time his vision returned to normal and his erection problems disappeared.

David was fortunate to have discovered his diabetes early and started treatment. His erection problem was temporary, caused by the high levels of blood glucose. He has realized that he can control his diabetes symptoms, including his erectile dysfunction, by keeping the blood glucose to a level of 140 mg/dl or less, which has become his goal.

Long-term erectile dysfunction

Diabetes can also cause erectile dysfunction that is long-lasting. The most common causes of this are damage to nerves and blockage of blood vessels by atherosclerosis. Diabetes can cause damage to nerve endings. This happens most commonly to the nerves in the legs, especially those that supply the feet and legs below the knees. You may feel tingling and numbness in the feet and lower legs, called *peripheral neuropathy*. This may also cause weakness of the muscles of the legs.

There may also be damage to the nerves that supply internal organs (autonomic neuropathy), including the organs of the pelvis, such as the stomach, bladder, and penis. It may be difficult to urinate as a result.

Nitric oxide is crucial for erections

The nerves to the penis are important in the release of nitric oxide, which is important in producing erections. Nitric oxide has been found by researchers to be low in these cases of nerve damage. With no nitric oxide, the small blood vessels which usually relax do not open to allow blood flow to increase in the penis. This is more often a long-lasting or permanent change that can limit erection. Nerve damage of this type is more common in smokers and in those over age 40.

> "If you have diabetes, make sure you know your A1c number. This test will show your average blood sugar level over the past 90 days. In contrast, your daily blood glucose testing only provides a snapshot of blood sugar control at that exact moment.
> —Caroline, endocrinologist, 35"

Case study illustrates importance of nitric oxide

Morris was 57 and had been diabetic for about 10 years. He maintained fairly good control of the blood glucose, although he found it hard to diet. Over the previous year he had noticed pins-and-needles sensations in his feet and legs in the areas that socks might cover. For a few months he had noticed his erections were not as full or long-lasting as they had always been, and on a few occasions this had caused him to be unable to complete his sexual activity.

Morris had a medical evaluation that found no other medical problems. He started back on his diet to manage his weight and to control blood glucose at near normal levels. With his doctor's recommendation, he began to take Viagra, and found that the quality of his erections greatly improved. Not only was he able to have erections that he felt were normal with a return to his usual sex life, but the erections lasted long enough to have satisfying sex.

Peripheral vascular disease can block erections

The other major problem that can create erectile dysfunction in diabetic men is peripheral vascular disease, which is atherosclerosis with hardening of the arteries in the legs. The blockage of the arteries lowers the amount of blood supply to the penis, so erections are limited. This may be difficult to treat unless the arterial circulation can be restored by surgery.

Case study illustrates problem firsthand

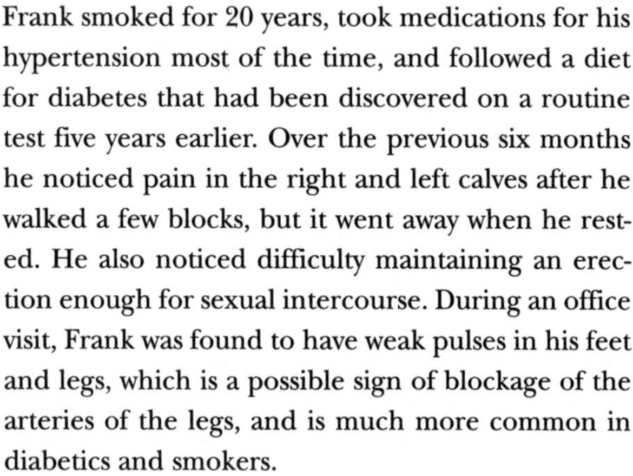

Frank smoked for 20 years, took medications for his hypertension most of the time, and followed a diet for diabetes that had been discovered on a routine test five years earlier. Over the previous six months he noticed pain in the right and left calves after he walked a few blocks, but it went away when he rested. He also noticed difficulty maintaining an erection enough for sexual intercourse. During an office visit, Frank was found to have weak pulses in his feet and legs, which is a possible sign of blockage of the arteries of the legs, and is much more common in diabetics and smokers.

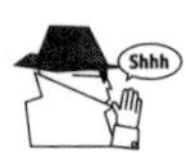

Unofficially... One out of every seven dollars spent on healthcare in the United States is spent on behalf of people with diabetes.

Further testing revealed that he had peripheral vascular disease caused by atherosclerosis. It was found to involve the arteries of the lower abdomen and pelvis as well as the legs, and caused the leg pain by limiting blood flow to the calf muscles when walking.

Steps were taken to help delay any worsening of the peripheral vascular disease and artery blockage. These included stopping cigarettes, and controlling the blood pressure and cholesterol levels. He also took aspirin daily, began a daily walking program, and tried Viagra for the erectile dysfunction. He noticed some improvement in erections with Viagra and also tried other treatments.

Other problems diabetics may face

Don't forget that diabetics can have any of the other problems that may cause erectile dysfunction.

These include low testosterone levels, stress-related problems that can severely limit erection, and side effects of medications given for other problems common in diabetics such as hypertension and heart disease. Check the list of risk factors for erectile dysfunction to be sure you don't blame a diabetic-related problem when it may be a separate cause, which is easily treatable.

In some diabetics there may be a combination of nerve damage and limitation of the artery supply of blood to the penis. Both of these problems are much more common in diabetics. This is the most difficult combination of problems to treat with medications.

Even in this situation, many treatments for erectile dysfunction are available.

Bright Idea
Ask your doctor about measuring the blood supply to your penis. Using a test called ultrasound, your doctor can tell the quality of the blood supply in the arteries and veins of the penis. There are also injections that can tell if the blood vessels are working well enough to allow an erection.

What about Viagra?

Viagra can be used if your doctor feels it is safe for you. If you have heart disease or you have had a stroke or ministroke (transient ischemic attack), then be sure you check with your doctor first. If you are taking any of the nitrate-related drugs such as nitroglycerin, you should not take Viagra because of the danger of sudden drops in blood pressure. In this situation one of the other treatments should be tried.

Remember that there is treatment available, it is simply a matter of which one is the best for you.

Control Is Crucial

Achieving control of blood glucose is the most important step you can take to ensure longevity, as well as regain control of your erections. With blood glucose monitoring and control, you can prevent complications such as:

- Eye damage (retinopathy)
- Nerve damage (neuropathy)
- Foot and leg problems
- Heart and blood vessel (cardiovascular) disease
- Impotence

> "The month before I was diagnosed with diabetes, I remember eating three hamburgers and two large colas for lunch and still being hungry. I ate like a horse but lost 15 pounds in three weeks."
> —Sam, attorney, 47

Your doctor will show you how to use electronic glucose monitoring, insulin pumps, and many other products, all designed to keep your blood sugar at normal levels. Staying on a healthy, balanced diet and exercising regularly are both crucial parts of your diabetic control.

Lose weight

If you are overweight, lose weight. Especially if you are an "apple" shape. Not only do men and women have different health concerns, they also gain weight in different places. For example, most women tend to gain in the hips and thighs, while men gain in the middle. The problem is that the apple shape is more at risk for diseases like diabetes than the pear shape. If you don't know whether your waist has expanded into a danger zone, then grab your measuring tape and calculate your waist/hip ratio, according to directions found in Table 5.1.

Obesity researchers are using waist/hip ratios to look at risks of developing different diseases. Men with waist/hip ratios greater than .95 are associated with increased risk of heart disease, high blood pressure, and diabetes. In fact, some researchers believe that from 50 to 75 percent of new cases of diabetes seem to be triggered by obesity.

TABLE 5.1: RECOMMENDED WAIST/HIP RATIO

Measure your waist (in inches), then divide this by your hip measurement (in inches over the widest part).

Women	Men
< .8	< .95

While researchers are not sure why being overweight increases the risk of diabetes, they do know from clinical studies that losing some weight helps control it. That came through loud and clear in a study of people at high risk for diabetes, who were overweight or whose parents had the disease. Researchers reported that these men and women cut their risk for diabetes by 30 percent simply by losing 10 pounds and keeping it off.

Move around more

Comprehensive research shows that from 30 to 50 percent of new diabetes cases diagnosed each year may be caused by too little exercise. Exercise can cut your risk of type 2 diabetes. Researchers believe that regular and ongoing exercise and activity such as walking, gardening, housework, playing with kids and grandkids, bowling, tennis, hiking, or any other enjoyable activity can make a significant difference for diabetics.

Exercise plays a key role in controlling blood glucose, yet in this case, the theory "no pain, no gain" is not valid. For the first time, research shows that light exercise—just as much as the heavy aerobic kind—reduces risk of developing diabetes.

Researchers at the University of South Carolina in Columbia studied 1,467 men and women aged 40 to 69. Some volunteers were healthy, others had a condition known as insulin resistance, the first step on the path to diabetes.

While researchers found that volunteers who spent the most time exercising gained the greatest level of diabetes protection, they also saw that people who walked or did other non-strenuous activities boosted their insulin sensitivity significantly.

These researchers concluded that diabetics and borderline diabetics who add moderate physical activity to their daily routines can help their bodies use insulin better and avoid serious consequences of this disease, such as amputation or blindness.

What activities might help you to avoid diabetes or at least control your blood sugar if you have diabetes? Try any exercises in Table 5.2 on a regular basis:

TABLE 5.2:
ACTIVITIES AND EXERCISES TO KEEP YOU HEALTHY

Badminton	Baseball	Basketball	Biking
Bowling	Dancing	Gardening	Golf
Handball	High-impact aerobics	Hiking	House cleaning
Karate	Kick boxing	Jumping rope	Low-impact aerobics
Mall walking	Mowing the yard	In-line skating	Rollerskating
Rowing	Running	Soccer	Softball
Stair-climbing	Stationary cycling	Strength training	Swimming
Tai Chi	Tae kwon do	Tennis	Vacuuming
Walking	Washing windows	Water exercises	Yoga

Dietary Control Is Possible

Diet plays such a crucial role, both in controlling blood glucose levels and in avoiding diabetes altogether. Staying on a finely calculated dietary plan that includes low-fat foods and controlled carbohydrates is crucial to good health.

Try carb counting

You've probably heard about the "exchange lists" diabetics have used in the past to plan their meals and control carbohydrates. While that method was appropriate and is even still used by many, there is a newer method of dietary control that gives more flexibility. This is called "carbohydrate counting"—or carb counting.

A carbohydrate is the name for sugars and starches in food. These substances directly affect blood sugar. With the newer method of carb counting, you keep track of the carbohydrates in your food.

For instance, scientific research shows that very little of the fat you eat is converted into glucose. Some of the protein you eat is converted into glucose, but it takes a long time. When you eat carbohydrates, within one hour more than 90 percent of this becomes glucose. For a diabetic, the increase in blood glucose comes from the carbohydrates you ate. Insulin balances glucose, so a good way to control blood glucose levels is to match your carbohydrates to insulin.

Carb counting will only work if you understand the principle and keep good records. You must test your blood glucose frequently throughout the day, record these levels, and measure the amount of carbohydrate eaten at each meal.

Make nutritional choices

There are numerous studies that show how foods and specific nutrients can alter blood sugar. One such study done by researchers at Brigham and Women's Hospital and Harvard Medical School found that vitamin C appears to dilate blood vessels and improve blood flow in diabetics.

Researchers gave vitamin C to 10 people with type 1 diabetes and to a similar group of volunteers without the diabetes. Scientists monitored blood flow in the volunteers' forearms and found that volunteers with diabetes had greater blood flow after taking vitamin C, while no change was found in the control group. Increasing blood flow to the extremities may help to prevent diabetes-related complications such as peripheral vascular disease that leads to amputation.

Another study by Dr. Emmanuel Opara and colleagues, of Duke University Medical Center in North Carolina, was presented at the Experimental Biology 98 meeting. Opara found that diabetics who eat a diet rich in antioxidants, such as vitamins C and E, may be able to slash their risk of complications such as amputation, blindness, and kidney failure.

Timesaver
If you want to learn more about carb counting, ask your doctor for a referral to a registered dietitian (RD) for counseling. Or, call the American Diabetes Association at (800) 232-3472.

These researchers studied 50 people with type 2 diabetes and 23 people without the disease. They were able to show that those with poor control of their diabetes and frequently had high blood sugar levels, and who were beginning to show signs of complications, had depleted their store of antioxidants. It appears that this deletion is a major risk factor for complications, and that antioxidant supplements may lower this risk.

Antioxidants neutralize free radicals, which are highly reactive—and harmful—oxygen molecules formed in the body through normal metabolic processes, and through such habits as smoking.

Look to low-fat foods

A common American diet contains more than 40 percent of the calories from fat. Since fats supply over twice as many calories per gram as carbohydrates or protein, we take in more calories, leading to weight gain.

While Americans are encouraged to reduce their intake of fats to no more than 30 percent of total calories, most people greatly exceed that figure. Many researchers point to this high-fat intake as causing a number of our chronic diseases, including obesity, which can lead to diabetes.

Think of the last time you indulged in a tender filet mignon, onion rings, and baked potato smothered in sour cream, then followed this gastronomical delight with a piece of New York cheese cake. This meal, while certainly appealing to many of us, provides more than 50 percent of its calories from fat and most of it is saturated!

Bright Idea
One way to know how many carbohydrates you have eaten is to look at the "Nutrition Facts" label on food packages. Nutritional labels list the number of grams of carbohydrate in one serving of that food.

Instead of eating like a bird to reduce excess weight, begin your daily menu plan with low-fat foods including vegetables, fruits, breads, whole grain cereals, legumes, fish, and skinless chicken. In controlled portions, these foods will allow you to feel full and still lose weight.

As you begin to look at your overall diet to reduce your weight and avoid or control diabetes, you are going to have to avoid the obvious high-fat foods:

- Fried chicken contains 55 percent fat.
- A fast food quarter-pound hamburger contains 55 percent fat.
- A fish fillet doubles its calories when bathed in butter and fried in oil.
- Cole slaw gets over 77 percent of its calories from fat.

Beware of the hidden fats

Fat can be easily recognizable in your diet in foods such as potato chips and sour cream dip, cheeseburgers and fries, and a bacon and egg breakfast. But some fats are dangerously hidden in seemingly healthy foods such as granola bars, peanut butter, cheese, some yogurts, popcorn cooked in oil, granola, and more. This is why everyone must become accustomed to reading labels and knowing the nutritional make-up of the foods they eat.

The recommended fat intake for one day is less than 30 percent of the total daily calorie intake. Many researchers and physicians, however, take this one step further and ask patients to lower their total daily fat intake to 20 to 25 percent or lower.

Making smart choices

While staying on a low-fat or no-fat diet seems out of reach for many of us, it can be done easily by making some choice substitutions in the daily diet. For example, by substituting skim milk for whole milk, reduced-fat margarine for butter, no-fat yogurt for regular yogurt, baked skinless chicken for fried chicken, and baked low-fat crackers or no-fat pretzels instead of fried chips. See Table 5.3 for more ways to reduce fat.

TABLE 5.3: WAYS TO REDUCE FAT IN YOUR DIET

Change This	To This
Ice cream	ice milk, sorbet, frozen yogurt
Butter	no-fat or reduced-fat margarine
Whole milk	low-fat or skim milk
Creamed soups	low-fat variety made with skimmed milk
French fries	baked oven fries
Potato chips	baked crackers or pretzels

Change This	**To This**
Cream	evaporated skim milk
Fried chicken	baked chicken without skin
Spaghetti sauce with meat	tomato sauce
Hamburger	grilled or broiled chicken sandwich
Candy bar	fudgsicle
Grilled cheese sandwich	grilled cheese with no-fat or low-fat cheese
Chocolate candy	no-fat jelly beans or candy corn
Omelet	egg substitutes or egg whites
Pancakes, biscuits, muffins	bagels, English muffins, rice cakes
Chocolate chip cookies	fig bars, gingersnaps
Pound cake	angel food cake
Regular mayonnaise	low-fat or no-fat mayonnaise
Tartar sauce	cocktail sauce or salsa
Cream cheese on bagel	no-fat cream cheese on bagel

To see if a food is high, moderate, or low in fat, it is important to read the label. Package labels include the ingredients, the calories, the fat content, nutrients, the sodium and fiber content, and much more for the consumer's information (see sample label).

TABLE 5.4: READ THE LABEL

Sample Label

Kraft Natural Finely Shredded Parmesan Cheese

Ingredients: Part-skim milk, cheese culture, salt, enzymes, aged over 10 months.

Nutrition Facts

Serving size 2 Tsp. (5 g)

Servings per container 17

Amount Per Serving

Calories 20

Calories from Fat 10

	% Daily Value*
Total Fat 1.5 g	2%
Saturated Fat 1 g	5%
Cholesterol less than 5 mg	1%
Sodium 75 mg	3%
Total Carbohydrate 0 g	0%
Dietary Fiber 0 g	0%
Sugars 0 g	
Protein 2g	
Vitamin A	0%
Vitamin C	0%
Calcium	4%
Iron	0%

Percent Daily Values are based on a 2,000 calorie diet. Your daily values may be higher or lower depending on your calorie needs.

Labels, however, can be confusing. Check out the list below:

- Low-fat means a product has no more than three grams of fat per serving.
- Low saturated fat means it has no more than one gram of saturated fat per serving.
- Reduced fat means the product has at least 25 percent less fat per serving than the traditional item.

- Light means the product has $^1/_2$ the fat or $^1/_3$ the calories of its regular counterpart.
- Fat-free has $^1/_2$ gram of fat or less per serving.

Calculating your fat calories

Trying to stay below 30 percent or an even more healthful 20 percent of fat calories each day means that you must carefully calculate this amount. After several weeks of doing this, it will become a "low-fat habit," and you will naturally turn to the healthier foods instead of unhealthy fat-laden choices.

If you eat 2,000 calories each day, you can calculate your fat calories by using the following formula:

2,000 calories × 30% fat calories = 600 calories from fat

You can now determine how many grams of fat allowed per day:

600 calories from fat ÷ nine calories per gram of fat = 66 grams of fat per day

Timesaver
After reading a label, you can quickly figure out the fat content by using the following formula:
1 gram fat = 9 calories
If the serving has 2 grams of fat, then
2 × 9 = 18 calories from fat
If the total calories for a serving are 100, then:
18÷100 = 18% of calories from fat

TABLE 5.5: FAT CONTENT OF SELECTED FOODS (BY PERCENTAGE OF CALORIES FROM FAT)

Foods with less than 30% fat		
Angel food cake	Bread	Fruits, all (with exceptions listed)
Chicken, roasted, light meat without skin	Pretzels	Rice
Cod fillets, broiled	Cottage cheese, 1% fat	Milk, 1% fat
Crab, cooked meat	Crackers, Saltines	Popcorn, plain
Dried beans and peas cooked without fat	Lentils	Pasta
Halibut fillets, broiled	Ice milk, vanilla	Sherbet, orange
Shrimp, steamed, shelled	Skim milk	Tuna, white (albacore) canned in water
Turkey, roasted, light meat without skin	Yogurt, plain, low-fat	Yogurt, fruit flavor, low-fat

Bright Idea
Try to stay below 30 percent or an even more healthful 20 percent of fat calories each day. This means that you must calculate the amount daily. Soon it will become a low-fat habit.

Foods with less than 30% fat		
Yogurt, frozen	Vegetables, all-with exceptions listed	Wheat germ

Foods with 30% to 40% fat		
Beef, rump lean only	Brownie, from mix	Flounder, fried
Cottage cheese, creamed (4% fat)	Flank steak	Granola
Ice milk, chocolate	Milk, 2% fat	Shrimp, fried
Turkey, roasted, dark meat without skin		

Foods with 40% to 50% fat		
Chicken, roasted dark meat without skin	Cookies, chocolate chip	Crackers, butter type
Chicken, roasted, light meat with skin	Cupcake with icing	Ice cream, vanilla
Milk, whole	Pork loin, lean, roasted	Salmon, canned
Tuna, white (albacore) canned in oil	Yogurt, whole milk	

Foods with 50% or more fat		
Avocado Bologna	Bacon	Beef rump roast, lean and fat
Butter	Cheeses, hard such as cheddar, Swiss	Coconut
Chicken, roasted, dark meat with skin	Cream cheese	Cream, table
Coffee creamer (containing palm oil), dry powder	Cream, half and half	Egg
Doughnut, cake-type	Doughnut, raised	Frankfurters
Ground beef	Margarine	Peanuts, roasted
Peanut butter	Pork loin, lean and fat	Salami
Sausage pork	Sour cream	

TABLE 5.6: FAT GRAMS

Calories Per Day	Grams of Fat 30% of calories	Grams of Fat 20% of calories
1000	33 grams	20 grams
1200	40 grams	24 grams
1500	50 grams	30 grams
1800	60 grams	36 grams
2000	67 grams	40 grams
2200	73 grams	44 grams
2400	87 grams	48 grams

Easy guidelines to reduce fat and obesity

The more serious you want to be about controlling fat in your diet, the closer you may want to follow these guidelines:

- Keep your fat intake to 30 percent or less of your daily caloric intake. You can easily do this by stocking *only* no-fat or low-fat items from the store. Why put temptation in front of you?
- Stay away from foods high in saturated fats (no more than 10 percent of your total calories per day).
- Choose your fats wisely. *No more* than 10 percent of your calories should come from polyunsaturated fat. Ten to 15 percent of your calories should come from monounsaturated fat (this is the "good" fat found in olive oil).
- Invest in a pocket-sized fat gram counter, and use it to look up the fat content of foods you regularly eat. Zero in on the highest-fat foods, and make some changes you can live with.
- Make subtle changes each week. Switching to skim milk instead of whole milk and eating skin-

"I've learned to substitute fat-free and low-fat sour cream, cream cheese, yogurt, ice milk, and milk for the high-fat versions. In making these subtle changes, I can still enjoy the taste and my weight has dropped by 10 pounds over the past six months.
—Wade, architect, 35"

less baked chicken instead of fried chicken could result in a reduction of calories—enough to lose 10 pounds in one year!

- Choose fish, skinned poultry, and lean red meat. Be sure to trim all visible fat from meat and poultry before cooking. When selecting cuts of meat, choose the "skinniest" cuts such as top round, tip round, sirloin, and chuck.
- Buy ground beef that is at least 90 percent lean or choose ground round or ground sirloin.
- Exchange ground turkey or chicken for part or even all of the beef in recipes for spaghetti, chili, meat loaf, or burgers. (Read the labels and buy ground white turkey or chicken, which has half the fat of dark meat).
- Avoid self-basting turkeys that are injected with heavy oils. Instead, use olive oil and defatted chicken or turkey broth for preparing a turkey.
- Buy water-packed tuna and save on fat calories while getting much-needed Omega-3s.
- Learn how to use tofu and legumes as meat substitutes. Have several "meatless" high-protein meals each week by combining legumes (e.g., red beans, navy beans, Great Northern beans) with pasta or rice. This meal will fill you up and is very low in fat.
- Use vegetarian refried beans in your tacos instead of meat filling. Make sure you check the label for the no-fat or low-fat variety.
- You can add low-fat ground turkey to red beans to make chili, or use beans instead of meat for spaghetti sauces.

- When choosing dairy products—go for the skim! Choose low-fat or no-fat cheeses, including cottage cheese, sour cream, cream cheese, yogurt, skim milk, and sugar-free ice milk. Also skim the broth for soups using defatted liquids. Canned undiluted skim milk for cream soups makes an excellent low-fat choice for mealtime.
- Instead of using a whole egg in a recipe, use two egg whites or egg substitute ($^{1}/_{4}$ cup equals one egg).
- To top your favorite berries, make fat-free whipped cream using chilled and whipped evaporated skim milk. Add one tablespoon lemon juice and sugar substitute; beat until stiff.
- Air popped popcorn and rice cakes make tasty fat-free snacks.
- Pretzels usually have one gram of fat per ounce (check label). This low-fat snack food has ten times less fat than chips.
- Use natural peanut butter with no oil or sugar added. Most grocery stores now carry peanut butter with less fat. Check your shelves.
- Watch the hidden calories in fast foods! That juicy hamburger contains over 50 percent of its calories in fat. Also be alert for high-fat menu terms such as "creamed," "sautéed," "au gratin," and "smothered."
- When ordering a main dish, request baked or broiled chicken or beef, and remember: extra crispy means extra calories!

Bright Idea
If you are looking for a breakfast meat that is not high in fat, choose Canadian bacon. It only has one gram of fat per ounce.

> "I used to order taco salads and think I was doing something low-fat and healthful until I read that the fried shell contains over 900 calories, and most of this is fat. Now I'm back to regular salads and a lot of vegetables—without added butter.
> —Stuart, stockbroker, 41"

- Instead of fries, choose a baked potato. But watch your toppings! They can be loaded with fat and calories, so heap on the tomatoes, mushrooms, broccoli, carrots, and cauliflower.
- Leave those high-fat toppings off pizza, and substitute onions, mushrooms, bell pepper, broccoli, and other vegetable toppings.
- Skip breakfast sandwiches for whole-grain cereal.
- Skip guacamole, sour cream, and refried beans when ordering Mexican foods. Choose tacos, tostados, or corn tortillas.

The following chart shows the most common oils and the varying fat content. Choose oils high in monounsaturated and polyunsaturated fats, and stay away from oils high in saturated fats.

TABLE 5.7: THE HEALTH DIFFERENCE IN OILS

Type of Oil	Saturated	Monounsaturated	Polyunsaturated
Safflower oil	9	13	78
Sunflower oil	11	20	69
Corn oil	13	25	62
Olive oil	14	77	9
Soybean oil	15	24	61
Peanut oil	18	48	34
Cottonseed oil	27	19	54
Lard	41	47	12
Palm oil	51	39	10
Beef tallow	52	44	4
Butterfat	66	30	4
Palm kernel oil	86	12	2
Coconut oil	92	6	2

Take Control Today

You know what to do, and now you know that control is up to you. If you are overweight, lose weight. Watch your fats and count your carbs, and move around more until you reach your normal weight. If you have diabetes, talk to a nutritionist about easy methods to control fluctuations in blood sugar levels. Most importantly, if you're tired a lot, have blurry vision, have lost weight for no reason, are thirsty all the time, and always have to go to the bathroom, you may have diabetes.

See your doctor to make sure you are free of this chronic disease, or call the American Diabetes Association for more information. The best way to prevent complications is with early intervention.

Just the Facts

- With blood glucose monitoring and control, you can prevent any complications, such as eye damage (retinopathy), nerve damage (neuropathy), foot problems, heart and blood vessel (cardiovascular) disease, and impotence.
- Eating a low-fat diet can help overweight adults reduce their weight, putting them at lower risk for type 2 diabetes.
- Controlling carbohydrates and balancing these with your blood glucose is crucial in staying well for diabetics.

Chapter 6

GET THE SCOOP ON...

How after age 35 the prostate gland can cause uncomfortable and even deadly problems ▪ The most common symptoms of prostatitis or prostate infection ▪ Which commonly used medication for enlarged prostate can cause impotence ▪ The consequences of early and late treatment of prostate cancer

The Threat of Prostate Disease

Everywhere you turn, you hear more and more news about the male prostate. This tiny gland is normally about the size of a walnut. It is important to your sexual health, secreting fluids to nurture the sperm during ejaculation.

While the prostate gland is silent most of your life, after age 35 it can make itself known in some uncomfortable and even deadly ways. The most common problems are infection, enlargement with blockage of urine flow, and prostate cancer, a cancer which can be deadly, if left untreated.

Checking Out the Prostate

The prostate gland is located below the pubic bone in front of the rectum at the base of the bladder (see Figure 6.1). The urethra is the tube that carries urine from the bladder to the penis. The urethra travels through the prostate gland, so an enlarged prostate gland may make passing urine difficult (see Figure 6.2).

The most common prostate concerns of most men are infection in the prostate (prostatitis), enlargement of the prostate, and cancer of the prostate.

FIGURE 6.1: MALE GENITALIA (SHOWING NORMAL PROSTATE/RECTUM/PUBIC BONE)

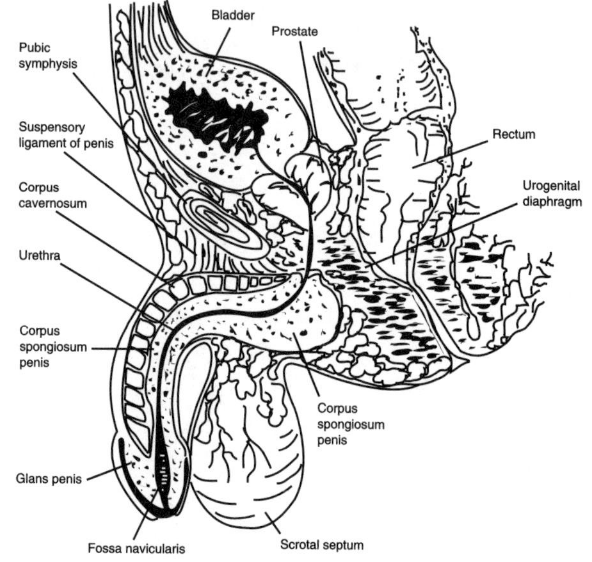

Prostatitis Can Interrupt Your Life

The most common symptom of prostatitis is an urgent sensation to urinate. Along with this urgency are the needs to urinate frequently and to get up at night to urinate, along with pain or burning when urinating. Many men report feeling discomfort such as fullness or pressure in the area between the scrotum and rectum. At times you might feel pain in the lower back. You probably won't notice any changes in the appearance of the urine, but it might appear cloudy.

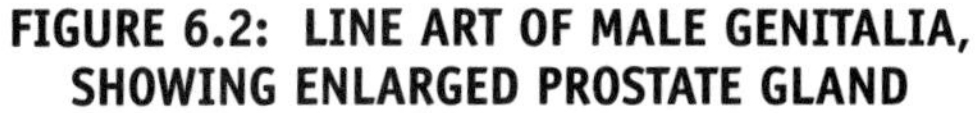

FIGURE 6.2: LINE ART OF MALE GENITALIA, SHOWING ENLARGED PROSTATE GLAND

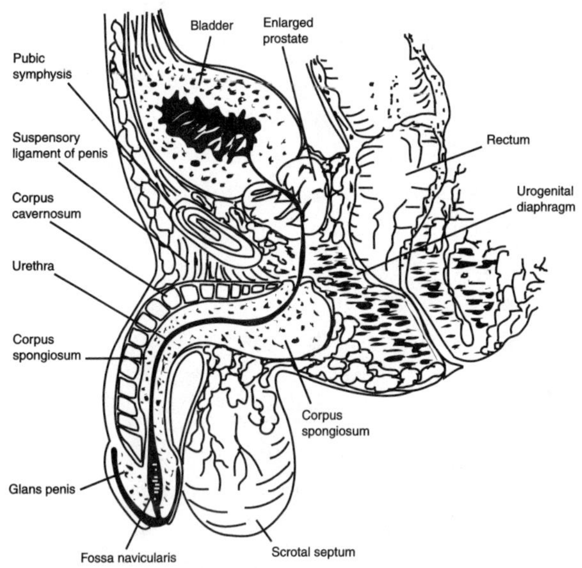

Making the diagnosis

Your doctor can tell if you have a prostate infection by a rectal exam of the prostate. Secretions from the prostate can be examined for changes typical of infection and cultures may prove the type of infection.

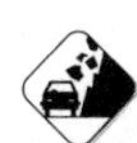

Watch Out!
Most antibiotic programs for treating a prostate infection will last for four to six weeks or longer. If antibiotics are used for shorter periods of time, it may be difficult to eradicate the infection. Be sure you take all your medicine, and let your doctor know if symptoms persist.

Treatment is not easy

Treatment for prostatitis, or a prostate infection, is with antibiotics, which must be taken for longer periods than you might take for most common infections.

Sitting in a warm bath for a few minutes once or twice a day may dispel feelings of discomfort and pressure until the antibiotic takes care of the infection.

Symptoms without infection

In many cases of prostatitis, no specific infection can be found. In these cases your doctor can ensure that no other more serious problems are causing the symptoms. You may need to see a urologist to be sure no other bladder or prostate disease is present.

> "For about six months I noticed a lower force of the urine stream, that eventually turned into a very weak stream. I also had dribbling at the end of urination. Finally, I asked my doctor, who checked my prostate. It was incredibly enlarged, but staying on medication for several months has lessened the symptoms dramatically.
> —Rick, teacher, 49"

In addition, your doctor may still try antibiotics for four weeks to be sure infection is not the cause. Prescription medications such as Minipres (prazosin), Hytrin (terazosin), or Cardura (doxazosin) are commonly used to control the irritating symptoms. Warm baths and ibuprofen may also help give relief.

The symptoms of this type of prostatitis may come and go over years. It helps to know that there are no other underlying serious complications from this common type of prostatitis. Your urologist can tell you if any further treatments would be helpful in your case.

Benign Prostatic Hyperplasia: A Non-cancerous Condition

BPH or benign prostatic hyperplasia (or hypertrophy) means an enlarged prostate gland, which is non-cancerous. When the gland is swollen, it presses against the urethra and makes urination painful and frequent. It may even interfere with the ability to completely empty the bladder.

The prostate becomes enlarged in practically all men at around age 35, and the increase in size continues gradually over a man's lifetime. Testosterone has a key role in this enlargement. A combination of aging and changes in hormones, specifically testosterone in the prostate changing into the more potent hormone DHT (dihydrotestosterone), is thought to cause BPH. In large concentrations, DHT causes cells to multiply and excessively enlarge the prostate.

What you may feel with BPH

As the enlargement of the prostate compresses the urethra, which carries urine from the bladder, you will begin to notice annoying symptoms.

Feeling the need to frequently urinate and frequent urination at night are typical of an enlarged prostate. This occurs because the bladder may not completely empty each time and needs to be emptied more often. Also, the prostate enlargement causes pressure on the bladder, sending a message that the bladder is full and needs to be emptied.

Furthermore, the muscle that empties the bladder may become more active and lead to more frequent urination. More nighttime urination is common since the muscles that keep the bladder from emptying are more relaxed while we sleep.

The symptoms that most men feel as the prostate enlarges and begins to cause obstruction are:

- Hesitation in starting the urine stream
- Weak or interrupted stream
- More frequent urination, especially during the night
- Infections in the bladder causing incomplete emptying

If you have any of these symptoms, tell your doctor. They may be caused by prostate enlargement or other serious medical problems. These problems can be prevented by early diagnosis and treatment.

Making the diagnosis

Your doctor will examine your prostate by a rectal exam. There are also other tests available to measure the size of the prostate. Your doctor may use a sonogram, which is safe and simple, and can provide an accurate measurement of the prostate. Your urologist will decide if any other tests are necessary.

Treating the enlarged prostate

There are many medications available for treating an enlarged prostate. With these medications, you can expect a good chance of improvement. Sometimes the medications can cause dizziness or heart palpitations. These same medications are used to treat hypertension, so some patients who have both problems may find relief in more than one area. If you don't have hypertension, the effect on the blood pressure is usually not a problem, but you need to be aware of this possible side effect. The most common of these medications are:

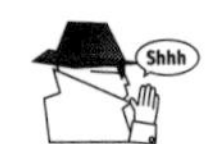

Unofficially... More than 50 percent of men over the age of 60 have benign prostatic hypertrophy and approximately 20 to 25 percent of those require treatment.

- Cardura
- Hytrin
- Proscar

Proscar (finasteride) is among a class of medications that works by suppressing the male hormones that stimulate the prostate enlargement. This medication has been found highly effective in more than half of patients who take it. In those who respond favorably to the drug, Proscar lowers the need for surgery and the risk of sudden blockage of urine. Hytrin (terazosin) and Cardura (doxazosin) work by relaxing the muscles in the bladder neck and prostate, which are often contracted and tighter than usual, and can obstruct urine flow.

Herbal treatments may work

Saw palmetto has been used for urinary and genital ailments for years. European studies have shown that the use of saw palmetto for three months seemed to decrease the frequency of nightly urination, while also decreasing the pain and difficulty with urination. Scientists suggest that the phytochemicals (naturally occurring plant chemicals) in saw palmetto berries help maintain a healthy prostate.

Another compound, beta-sitosterol, is found naturally in soybeans, pumpkin seeds, and palmetto berries, and may also help to keep your prostate healthy. These phytochemicals are similar in structure to testosterone and estrogen and may block the receptor sites of these hormones and limit their effect on the prostate. Vegetarians consume more of these beneficial compounds than do meat eaters.

Watch Out! Proscar (finasteride) can occasionally cause lowering of libido or erectile dysfunction, so be aware of this possibility. Also, the result of the blood test for PSA may be lower while taking Proscar, but this should not affect your doctor's ability to check for prostate cancer.

When surgery is warranted

When medicines are not effective, surgery is the next step in treating benign prostatic hyperplasia. The following surgical techniques are commonly used:

- TURP (transurethral resection of the prostate) is the most commonly used procedure. In this operation, the part of the prostate gland that is causing the blockage is removed by inserting an instrument into the penis. Part of the enlarged prostate is then removed through the urethra. This is usually done with spinal anesthesia, nerve block, or general anesthesia. The operation is quite safe, though some studies show 20 to 30 percent of patients may have a complication of some type. Urinary retention is uncommon, but it can occur.

- A transurethral incision of the prostate can be performed instead of TURP. In this procedure, small incisions are made in the prostate gland near the bladder. This method is used if you have symptoms of blockage, but the prostate gland is not very enlarged.

- The enlarged prostate can also be removed by an operation with an incision above the pubic bone. This is usually done when the prostate gland is very large and requires a longer recovery than TURP.
- Laser surgery to remove the enlarged prostate is becoming more widely used. This type of surgery has fewer complications initially and takes less time, but some patients develop urinary retention after surgery (i.e., the bladder does not empty). This side effect lasts longer than it does with TURP. Patients sometimes need a second operation later. Newer laser techniques may offer results comparable to TURP surgery with fewer complications.

Bright Idea
If you decide to try saw palmetto, be sure to find a product that is standardized to provide 85 to 95 percent phytoesterols. Other products, including pygeum and stinging nettle, are not as well-studied for treatment of BPH as saw palmetto.

- Transurethral evaporation of the prostate uses a high-power density beam in an instrument inserted into the urethra to eliminate prostate tissue.
- Balloon dilatation of the prostate inflates a balloon to expand the diameter of the urethra in the prostate area. This procedure may require the use of prostate stents—metal coils that are inserted into the urethra to keep it open. These are good in cases where surgery may not otherwise be advisable.
- Microwave hyperthermia uses heat to damage prostate cells, which are then eliminated. This is an outpatient procedure that does not require surgery and may give relief of prostate symptoms in most patients.

- High-intensity ultrasound uses ultrasound to produce heat and damage the prostate tissue, which then becomes smaller, hence relieving symptoms.
- Treatment with high frequency radio waves is done by Transurethral Needle Ablation (TUNA), which reduces the size of the enlarged prostate tissue. The treatment is delivered through the urethra by an antenna. This is less invasive than surgery and can be done as an outpatient.

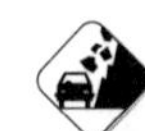

Watch Out!
Medications such as Proscar and Hytrin are approved for treatment of enlarged prostate, although each has negative side effects such as impotence and a decreased sex drive (Proscar) and dizziness and low blood pressure (Hytrin). Surgery is effective but also has risks of leaving you incontinent or impotent.

Every Man's Fear: Prostate Cancer

Prostate cancer is the second leading cause of cancer death in American men, with about 200,000 cases diagnosed each year. This type of cancer is rare before age 40, more common after age 50, and is said to strike nearly one in 10 men. Studies show that if a man lives to the age of 80, his chances of getting prostate cancer rise to one in three.

In fact, prostate cancer may be present in as many as 75 percent of men over age 75. However, this cancer often goes undiscovered during life, which means it is small and slow-growing.

The important thing to remember about prostate cancer is that it can be cured when found early. Interestingly, unlike many cancers, prostate cancer may have a good outlook even without treatment, depending on the type of cancer cells involved. This has led many researchers to question giving aggressive treatment, especially to older men, which may have serious side effects such as impotence and urinary incontinence.

What you may feel

The following is a list of the common symptoms of prostate cancer:

- Difficulty with urination
- Frequency of urination
- Pain with ejaculation
- Blood in the urine
- Blood with ejaculation

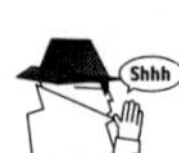

Unofficially... You may be at higher risk for prostate cancer if you have a family member who was affected. African-Americans have a higher chance of prostate cancer than white men.

However, there is no need to wait for symptoms to appear. Today, screening tests, especially the routine PSA blood test (Prostate Specific Antigen) and the rectal exam of the prostate uncover most cases of prostate cancer.

The PSA blood test has created much interest because it can detect prostate cancer by as much as 11 years earlier than by other methods or with no testing at all.

Making the diagnosis

While studies show that 70 percent or more patients with prostate cancer have high PSA test levels, BPH or a non-cancerous infection can also cause elevated PSA.

The biggest problem is telling the difference between an abnormal PSA from cancer and an abnormal PSA from other causes.

Researchers have now found that there are different forms of PSA in the blood. The PSA of prostate cancer patients is carried on other proteins, while that of BPH circulates alone or free. Measuring the amount of *free* PSA can give your doctor a more accurate prediction of whether a high PSA is from prostate cancer. This increases the chances of early detection.

What's normal; what's not

The normal levels of PSA are usually 0 to 4 ng/ml, and about 25 percent of patients with PSA above 4 will have prostate cancer. Researchers have found, however, that PSA may increase slightly with age, so in older patients, high PSA may not indicate cancer. If your tests reveal high PSA, knowing how your PSA relates to your age and family history of prostate cancer will help your doctor determine if a biopsy is required. Taking this age factor into account may help you avoid an unnecessary biopsy.

If your PSA is high but no cancer is found, your doctor may follow with repeat tests at six- to 12-month intervals, because PSA in patients with prostate cancer may increase faster than those with only BPH.

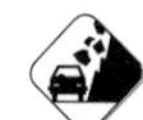

Watch Out!
If you are taking saw palmetto and due for a PSA test (Prostate Specific Antigen test), tell your health care professional, as the results of your test could be affected.

One early sign of prostate cancer is a small lump on the prostate. If a rectal exam discovers a nodule, your urologist may order a sonogram of the prostate. Using the results of this test your urologist may ask for a simple biopsy of the prostate, which is the only way to make an accurate diagnosis. If prostate cancer is found, the tests will tell the tumor grade, which is a measure of the chances that the tumor will grow quickly or slowly. This is one of the most useful predictors of the future growth of the prostate cancer.

The prostate tumor's stage tells the size and spread of the tumor. This allows your urologist to predict how the prostate cancer might behave in the future. A CT (computed tomography) scan, MRI (magnetic resonance imaging), or bone scan are used along with the prostate sonogram to decide the stage of the prostate cancer. At times, biopsies of lymph nodes around the prostate in the pelvis are taken. Together, this information helps your urologist plan the best possible treatment for the prostate cancer.

The best methods of treatment

If the cancer is early and localized, surgery to remove the prostate (radical prostatectomy) or radiation therapy are the two most common treatments.

Bright Idea
Just as most women do monthly breast self-examinations, men should perform monthly testicular self-examinations. The easiest time to perform this is when you are taking a shower. Using both hands, examine each testicle with the thumbs in front. Place your first two fingers behind the testicle. Roll the testicle between your thumb and fingers to see if there are any lumps or hard spots.

With radical prostatectomy, the prostate is removed from above the pubic bone or between the scrotum and rectum. This surgery can cause incontinence, with leakage of urine varying from one to 11 percent, but averaging about five percent.

Erectile dysfunction happens in about 25 percent of cases and is less with newer surgery which protects the nerves that supply the penis.

Radiation therapy is the other major treatment for early prostate cancer. This type of treatment takes six to seven weeks by external beam radiation therapy, which is directed at the prostate to destroy cancer cells. Radiation therapy using radioactive implants is also possible. Intestinal problems, including rectal bleeding, diarrhea, and abdominal pain, and other problems occur in up to 20 percent of cases. Twenty-five to 80 percent of men develop impotence with erectile dysfunction after radiation therapy. Erection problems may develop months after the treatment is completed. About 10 percent of patients experience difficulty urinating, and painful or frequent urination, although this side effect is usually not permanent.

For more advanced prostate cancer, other effective treatments are available. Your urologist can guide you. Treatments available include:

- Hormone treatment with estrogens, which stop the production of testosterone and therefore remove its effect on the prostate cancer cells.

- Removal of the testicles (orchiectomy), which also removes testosterone and its effect on the cancer.
- Newer hormone treatments that reduce testosterone and stop the production of the hormones that stimulate the testicles.
- A combination of treatments, including the use of more than one type of medication.

Advanced cancer hinders treatment

As prostate cancer becomes more advanced, treatment becomes more complicated and less effective. Early detection and treatment are therefore crucial. This means yearly testing for men over 50, beginning earlier if you are at higher risk.

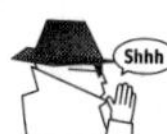

Unofficially... Testicular cancer is the most common cancer in men from age 18 to 34.

Testicular Cancer

Prostate cancer is not the only cancer found only in men. Testicular cancer is another common cancer. However, when detected early, this type of cancer is one of the most easily cured.

If testicular cancer is not diagnosed and treated at an early stage, it may spread throughout the lymph node system into the lungs and remaining parts of the body. Unfortunately, testicular cancer can be especially dangerous because there are often no symptoms associated with it.

What you may feel

Testicular cancer starts as a small pea-sized lump within the testicle. You may notice this lump during your regular monthly testicular self-examinations. If you don't perform these routinely, the chances are great that you might miss this diagnosis.

Keep in mind, if you do find a lump, it may not mean cancer. Not all swellings or lumps in the scrotum are cancer. Nonetheless, if you find a pea-sized lump, call your doctor and get it checked.

Your testicle should normally feel similar to a hard-boiled egg without the shell. If lumps or bumps are discovered, contact your doctor. Keep in mind that the best form of prevention and staying cancer-free is early diagnosis and treatment.

Making the diagnosis

Tremendous advances have been made, not only in diagnosis, but also in treatment of testicular cancer. In addition to specific blood tests that are now available to detect testicular cancer, sound waves can make a visual image of the testicle and reveal any abnormalities.

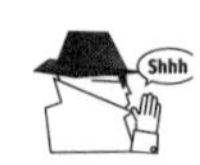

Unofficially... About 300,000 operations are performed each year to treat enlarged prostate.

Protecting Yourself from Colon Cancer

According to the American Cancer Society, an estimated 67,600 men were diagnosed with colon cancer in 1996. Of these cases, about 27,400 will die of their disease. In the past three decades, the mortality rates for women diagnosed with colon cancer have fallen 31 percent. The mortality rates for men have dropped by only 9 percent.

Know the warning signs

Warning signs of colon cancer include rectal bleeding, blood in the stool, or a change in bowel habits. Most often, however, colon cancer has no symptoms until it's too late. The American Cancer Society recommends a stool blood test and a sigmoidoscopy after the age of 50 to detect colon cancer even if no symptoms are present. These tests offer the best opportunity to remove polyps before they become cancerous.

Understanding flexible sigmoidoscopy

Flexible sigmoidoscopy is a visual examination of the lining of the rectum and a portion of the colon using a lighted, flexible, fiber-optic tube about the thickness of your finger. This remarkable piece of equipment can be directed and moved around the bends in the lower colon and rectum.

Avoidance keeps many men from having a flexible sigmoidoscopy. Yet this simple outpatient exam takes only 10 minutes and provides the physician with a great deal of useful information. The exam is performed while lying on your side in a comfortable position. The procedure should be painless, although you may feel slight pressure or a bloated sensation.

When colon cancer is detected early, before it spreads to other parts of the body, the five-year survival rate is 91 percent. However, when the cancer is not caught in time, five-year survival rates drop to 63 percent.

Watch Out!
Colon cancer is most often detected in men who have a personal or family history of colorectal cancer polyps, or inflammatory bowel disease. Other factors that put you at risk include physical inactivity and a high-fat diet and/or a low-fiber diet.

Kidney Stones—Another Common Problem in Men

Kidney stones are a common problem, especially with men. These rock-like pebbles are caused by an abnormal formation of deposits in the kidney and create painful blockages, preventing the flow of urine out of the body.

A kidney stone may be as tiny as a pencil eraser or even the head of a pin, or as large as a marble or the size of a golf ball. They are not perfectly round in shape, but are irregular with sharp projections.

The pain produced by a kidney stone can be excruciating and can be felt intensely in the lower back.

While the majority of kidney stones (about 85 percent) are made up of calcium, there are also stones composed of uric acid and ammonium.

What you may feel

The stone will not cause you pain when it rests in the kidney. However, as soon as the stone drops into your ureter (the tube that carries the urine from the kidney to the bladder), the obstruction and resulting swelling cause extreme pain.

Making the diagnosis

If your doctor suspects you may have a kidney stone, after evaluating the urine for blood by urinalysis, you may be referred to have an IVP (intravenous pyelogram) x-ray. This type of x-ray will help your doctor determine the exact location and size of the stone, as well as if multiple stones are present.

How they are treated

You may pass the stone without any medical assistance—85 percent of people do—but only if it is small enough to move through the ureter without getting stuck. If your stone is larger, be glad that the treatment of kidney stones has been much improved over the past decade. Some of the most common ways to zap kidney stones include:

- Extra Corporeal Shock Wave Lithotripsy (ESWL)—a new treatment option that sends sound waves into the body. These waves "bomb" or fragment the stone into fine particles that are then passed out with the normal flow of urine.
- Ureteroscopy—a treatment involving the passage of a long, thin telescope up through the ureter to where the stone is located. The stone may then be zapped with a laser or an ultrasonic probe.
- Indirect manipulation and extraction of the stone with wires and baskets.

Prevent Serious Problems Altogether

We all do what we can to take care of our heart. But all men should also make prevention of prostate and related genital problems, including cancer, an optimal health goal. It is now known that most of those who suffer from male genitalia problems can benefit greatly from lifestyle changes, including regular exercise, quitting cigarettes, avoiding too much alcohol, staying at a normal weight, and eating a low-fat diet, among many others.

The main ingredient in the treatment and prevention of cancers specific to men is *you*. Start becoming aware of the warning signs of the serious problems addressed in this chapter, then talk with your doctor about preventive measures. Be sure to do monthly self-examinations to catch problems like testicular cancer early, when treatment is most effective. In other words, in this day and age, any man can change his life so that the chances of dying from male cancers are greatly reduced.

It's in your court!

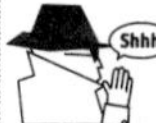

Unofficially... Only uric acid stones have been found to be dissolvable with medication. However, increasing the amount of fluids you drink and reducing the amount of calcium supplements can prevent kidney stones.

Just the Facts

- Frequent, hesitant, or weak urination may indicate an enlarged prostate.
- Although prostate cancer is rare before age 40, it is the second leading cause of cancer in men.
- One side effect of surgery for prostate cancer is impotence.

Chapter 7

GET THE SCOOP ON...

The widespread consequences of snoring and obstructive sleep apnea (OSA) ▪ How OSA can lead to hypertension, stroke, and even death ▪ The treatment for OSA ▪ Polysomnography, "pure" snoring, and OSA

The Unknown Perils of Obstructive Sleep Apnea

Most of us know that staying young, feeling energetic, and being productive is the quintessential goal to compete in today's world. While we cannot stop the clock, we can stop problems commonly associated with aging, such as snoring or obstructive sleep apnea, which can rob you of precious sleep, vitality, youthfulness—as well as your ability to perform sexually.

Snoring is a universal complaint that affects more than 40 million men and women (and their bed partners, family members, and co-workers). Not only can nighttime snoring make you feel exhausted the next day, it is associated with such problems as memory loss, depression, hypertension, cardiovascular disease, stroke, and impotence.

What Is Snoring?

Snoring is a very common low-frequency noise that occurs during sleep. It is the direct result of airflow limitation and the associated vibration of the soft tis-

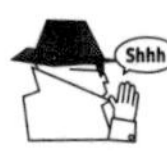

Unofficially... While more than 60 percent of all men ages 35 to 65 snore, women are not immune. In fact, more than 40 percent of all women ages 35 to 65 snore. This is a number that soars dramatically at menopause. Snoring sometimes diminishes in men after age 65, yet it remains stable in women.

sues in the back of the throat. It can also be a symptom of a very serious medical condition called obstructive sleep apnea (OSA), which involves severe narrowing or occlusion of the airway, which can cause a pause in breathing.

With OSA, your lungs do not get enough air so the brain wakes you up just enough to catch your breath and unblock the air passage. You may experience frequent sleep interruptions, along with choking or gasping spells upon waking.

The condition is so subtle that you may not even realize that you were aroused from sleep, yet when this occurs many times during the night, the results are poor sleep, reduced oxygen in the body, and daytime sleepiness. In fact, in many cases, it is your bed partner who tells you of the sleep apnea episodes and becomes frightened because of your inability to breathe. OSA can also lead to severe cardiac and pulmonary problems, even to death. Little do millions of men realize that one of the symptoms of OSA is impotence.

Snoring snuffs out sex

While the snorer may sleep seemingly undisturbed by his own nocturnal noises, sound levels of snoring have been recorded as high as 88 decibels—as loud as the diesel engine one hears when sitting in the back of an old bus. Not only are these nocturnal sounds an annoying nuisance to the sleepless bed partner, but snoring can interrupt one's sexual relationship. Studies have consistently revealed that men who snore heavily and have the associated OSA lose their sexual urges and are faced with impotence. For their bed partners, how sexy is it to lie in bed and listen to your mate continually make thunderous roars, gasps, and sighs throughout the night, then suffer with the consequences of sleep loss, daytime fatigue, and an inability to concentrate on love making?

More than 42 percent of men with OSA are impotent. Studies have consistently revealed that men who snore heavily and have OSA may lose their sexual urges because of fatigue and/or depression just as some depressed people lose their appetite for food. Problems maintaining a penile erection can be the result of fatigue or coincidental vascular and/or neurologic abnormalities seen in men who have OSA. These men may also be older or have other medical problems, such as high blood pressure, or diabetes mellitus. Some men taking medications for hypertension or depression may experience impotence. Treatment of OSA, a possible underlying cause of the high blood pressure or depression, may get rid of or reduce the need for these drugs and improve sexual function.

Not for men only

In one study performed in Ontario, Canada, 86 percent of the women questioned said their mates snored. Interestingly, more than 57 percent of the men said their wives snored.

Not only is snoring shared by both sexes, it is an extremely serious social and public health hazard. This medical problem causes poor quality of sleep, changes in the sleep/wake cycle, and lower levels of oxygen in the blood as a result of OSA. Because of restless sleep and frequent awakenings, there is diminished daytime alertness resulting in dramatic alterations in mood, effectiveness, and energy.

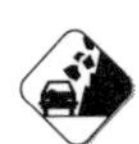

Watch Out!
Did you know that waking up during the night to go to the bathroom is also correlated with snoring? If you have to frequently urinate at night, ask your doctor if a sleep study would help diagnose snoring or obstructive sleep apnea. Seeking treatment for these ailments may help you sleep through the night—without awakening at all.

A costly condition

Poor sleep and the resulting daytime sleepiness and mental impairment caused by snoring are also expensive, costing companies billions of dollars from:

- Reduced productivity
- Increased motor-vehicle accidents
- Increased coronary artery disease and heart attacks
- Increased accidental injuries and deaths at work
- Increased medical and psychiatric illnesses
- Increased employee turnover

A new health concern

Interestingly, when the first medical book on sleep disorders was published in 1968, snoring was only addressed on 22 pages. Until that time, most scientists assumed that while snoring was an annoying nuisance, it was simply a natural occurrence of aging. There were no sleep studies or hints that snoring could actually cause heart disease, stroke, or even death.

Today we know differently. In the early 1970s, epidemiological studies began to reveal startling evidence that snoring was *far more* than a noisy distraction. Through a number of scientific studies, it became clear that a host of serious health problems are much more frequent among habitual snorers.

So much myth and lack of information surround snoring that many people are shocked to find out that snoring is correlated with the extra girth accumulated through the years. It is also associated with high blood pressure. Millions of men who suffer with erectile dysfunction are astounded when the urologist links their impotence with something as seemingly benign as nighttime snoring.

A 45-year-old man who awakened frequently to urinate was convinced he had prostate disease until a sleep study confirmed OSA. Another middle-aged man, who also suffers with nasal rhinitis and asthma, could not believe that his continual snoring was the reason he could no longer think clearly, remember names, or concentrate at work. He had worried for months that this was the first stage of Alzheimer's disease until he received the diagnosis of "snoring" and the subsequent cure.

Pure Snoring or Obstructive Sleep Apnea?

As stated, snoring may be an early warning sign for OSA. Snoring is caused by the vibration of the soft parts of the throat while inhaling air during sleep, and this noise may be continuous with almost every breath or intermittent with breath-holding spells. These periods of suspension of breathing are called apneas, which are due to obstruction of the upper airway at the level of the uvula, which hangs down from the back of the roof of the mouth, or base of the tongue. Apneas may be interrupted by a brief arousal that can be recorded from brain waves in a sleep disorder laboratory.

In adults, *10 to 50 percent of those who snore have sleep apnea.* Why the wide range of figures? Millions of those who snore have not been diagnosed with this serious problem, yet have the serious symptoms. In fact, in adults, OSA is more common than asthma. Those with more than 20 apneas (complete obstructions) per hour of sleep may have a greater

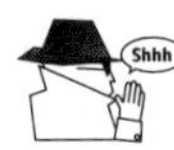

Unofficially... Those with obstructive sleep apnea not only snore but often have other very serious symptoms after what they thought was a good night's sleep, as the arousals fragment or ruin the normally refreshing nature of sleep. Low oxygen levels, which result when the blockages prevent air from getting to the lungs, also affect brain and heart function.

risk of dying than people with fewer apneas. Up to two-thirds of the people who have OSA are overweight. Analysis of data from several studies suggests that the association among snoring and high blood pressure, coronary disease, and strokes may be due to obesity and the presence of OSA.

Problems resulting from OSA

Problems or medical complications associated with untreated sleep apnea may include:

- Systemic hypertension—High blood pressure that causes an increased risk of heart disease, strokes, kidney failure, and poor circulation.
- Left-side heart failure—Inability of the heart to pump the blood adequately, causing shortness of breath, fatigue, and poor ability to exercise.
- Pulmonary hypertension—Elevated blood pressure in the lungs, associated with shortness of breath, chest pain, and increased mortality.
- Arrhythmias—Irregularity of the heart beat.
- Ischemic heart disease—Angina pectoris (chest pain) and heart attacks (myocardial infarction) caused by an insufficient supply of blood to the heart.
- Stroke—Damage to the brain caused by blockage of blood flow or bleeding.
- Early mortality
- Excessive daytime sleepiness (EDS)
- Impaired daytime performance
- Personality changes

Getting a diagnosis

Do you want to be haunted your entire lifetime by this irritating, roaring whistle that flows out of your throat during sleep? Of course not! Does your bed partner relish staying awake night after night, poking you in the side in the hope you will quit? We doubt it! Or, has your partner already moved to another room at the other end of your home to avoid being awakened? Probably! Then maybe it's time to head to your doctor for an accurate diagnosis and effective treatment.

Identifying symptoms

Measure your daytime sleepiness on the Epworth Sleepiness Scale (Table 7.1), and assess the chance you have of dozing each day in specific situations.

Some sleep medicine experts use the Epworth Sleepiness Scale to evaluate a person's tendency to doze off during the day. The Epworth Sleepiness Scale involves assigning a number to the likelihood of falling asleep in certain circumstances such as sitting and reading, watching television, or as a passenger in a car for more than an hour. A total score above seven is considered abnormal. The higher the score, the more likely you will doze off.

After you measure your sleepiness, check out Table 7.2 and see which symptoms you might have for OSA. Write these down, and let your doctor know at the consultation.

How likely are you to doze off or fall asleep during the day in the following situations, as opposed to feeling just tired? This refers to your recent, usual way of life. Use the following scale to choose the most appropriate number for each situation. A total score above seven is considered abnormal, and the higher the score the more likely you will doze off.

TABLE 7.1: THE EPWORTH SLEEPINESS SCALE

Would never doze	0
Slight chance of dozing	1
Moderate chance of dozing	2
High chance of dozing	3
Situation	Chance of Dozing
Sitting and reading	_____
Watching television	_____
Sitting, inactive in a public place (for example, in a theater or meeting)	_____
Lying down to rest in the afternoon	_____
Sitting and talking with someone	_____
Sitting quietly after lunch without alcohol	_____
In a car, while stopped for a few minutes in traffic	_____

TABLE 7.2: COMMON SYMPTOMS OF OBSTRUCTIVE SLEEP APNEA

Morning headaches	High blood pressure	Dry mouth
Sore throat upon awakening	Depression	Memory failure
Concentration problems	Impotence	Irregular heart rhythm

The following is a list of the common risk factors for OSA:

- Gender: Males twice as common as females
- Obesity: Greater than 120% ideal body weight
- Neck Size: Collar greater than 17 inches in men and 15 inches in women
- Enlarged tonsils
- Nasal septum deviation, which causes difficulty when breathing through the nose
- Small jawbone or backward displacement of jawbone

- Glandular disorders: Hypothyroidism, acromegaly
- Genetic predisposition: Family history

Medicines or drugs may worsen snoring or cause OSA. These include:

- Alcohol
- Hypnotics (sleeping pills)
- Narcotic pain relievers
- Tranquilizers

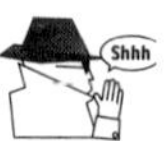

Unofficially... A respiratory disturbance index (RDI) may be calculated to assess the severity of abnormal respiratory events, based on their frequency. The RDI gives the number of abnormal respiratory events per hour of sleep.

Sleep studies confirm diagnosis

To clinch the diagnosis of OSA, your doctor will recommend special sleep studies. Polysomnography can provide an important assessment of the occurrence of apneas, measures of oxygenation during sleep, and electrocardiographic abnormalities. These tests also measure the severity of sleep fragmentation such as arousal, sleep-stage shifts, or shortage of REM sleep. These tests can also detect other sleep disorders that may be contributing to the excessive daytime sleepiness. Recordings taken during a sleep study include:

- Electroencephalography—uses special electrodes or probes placed on the scalp for recording electrical activity from the brain.
- Electrooculogram—records the electrical voltage that exists between the front and back of the eye. This particular electrical activity changes along with eye movement and is detected by electrodes placed on the skin near the eye.
- Electromyogram—involves an instrument that converts electrical activity associated with functioning muscle into a written or visual record.

Airflow at your nose and mouth, respiratory effort, oxygen levels, leg movements, and body position (supine, prone, side) are also recorded. An electrocardiogram is also taken. A sleep study should include a sufficient amount of REM and non-REM sleep.

If you have snoring but no evidence of other symptoms, overnight oximetry (oxygen level monitoring) during sleep in your home may be helpful as a screening tool. If the test shows a significant pattern of oxygen drops, a full polysomnogram then may be warranted for a definitive diagnosis.

Finding Treatment That Works

Once the diagnosis of pure snoring or OSA has been confirmed, your doctor will make sure that you understand the health risks associated with this disorder. Problems such as an increased tendency to suffer from high blood pressure, abnormal heart rhythms, strokes, and heart attacks are all attributed to sleep apnea.

The excessive daytime sleepiness itself may cause major complications because impaired alertness can cause accidents in your job or during travel. Your performance at the office or in social settings can also suffer from daytime sleepiness. You need to comprehend the risks of this condition and also the effectiveness of the various treatment methods that are available. Choice of therapy needs to be made based on the specific nature and severity of the sleep apnea in each case.

Specially made dental appliances such as the Herbst prosthesis may be used to pull the jawbone forward to widen the airway space at the base of the tongue. Some people have found excellent results with nasal dilators purchased at any grocery or drug store, combined with a nasal decongestant spray to open blocked airways.

If your doctor diagnoses you with "pure" snoring, that is, snoring without OSA, the options for treatment are many. Check out the following treatments for snoring, and see which will work in your situation.

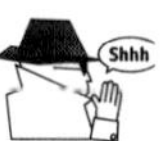

Unofficially... Obesity is defined as being 20 percent or more over normal body weight. It affects one-third of the U.S. population. On the other hand, even being slightly overweight may also contribute to your snoring problem.

Lose weight

While there are many ways to cure snoring, both surgically and non-surgically, losing weight is often the best way to guarantee that the cure will work. In fact, studies show that gaining weight after having surgery for sleep apnea could worsen the problem. When snoring or OSA is combined with obesity, it becomes a dangerous issue. It only takes a quick glance in the mirror to know if you would benefit from losing a few pounds. Men may not need to look into a mirror as some experts believe an expanding neck measurement says it all, especially for those who have fat stores around their neck. If you are a male, and your neck is a size 17 or larger and has increased over the years, chances are, so has your girth, adding to your problem with snoring.

Not only does carrying around extra baggage increase your snoring, weighing as little as 10 or 15 pounds over your desired weight can exacerbate a heart condition, elevate blood pressure and cholesterol, and even increase your risk of certain cancers. In the midst of the pessimistic outlook for overweight individuals, there is some good news. While gaining weight can increase the chance of snoring, as well as serious illness, losing weight can reduce the risk.

While height/weight charts used to give an accurate range, newer studies show that your body mass index (BMI) seems to give a more accurate picture of health. According to the American Dietetic Asso-

Watch Out!
While older forms of antihistamines get into the brain and cause drowsiness, newer forms do not do this. For this reason, if you have sleepiness due to obstructive sleep apnea, you need to avoid the older, sedating antihistamines.

ciation, people with a higher percentage of body fat tend to have a higher BMI than those who have a greater percentage of muscle. It is this extra body fat, not muscle, that puts you at greater risk for health problems.

Using the BMI chart (see Figure 7.3), locate your weight along the left-hand column, then slide your finger across the top until you come to the number nearest your height. Where these two columns meet is your BMI. For example, if you weigh 180 pounds and are 5' 8" tall, your BMI is 27, or not at high risk for chronic illness such as OSA. Table 7.3 gives you an idea of how healthy—or unhealthy—your BMI is. Keep in mind that each of us is different. Your weight can depend on many variables, including your height, age, and bone structure. The best weight for you is the one where you are healthy and, hopefully, do not snore!

TABLE 7.3: BMI INDEX

BMI	Risk for Health Problems Related to Body Weight
20-25	Very low risk
26-30	Low risk
31-35	Moderate risk
36-40	High risk
40+	Very high risk

End nasal congestion

Nasal congestion can easily add to your snoring problem. Do you know whether to take an antihistamine or decongestant when you have nasal congestion? It depends on your symptoms and the exact triggers of your nasal problem.

FIGURE 7.1: BODY MASS INDEX (BMI)

	Body Mass Index (BMI) Height (ft, in)																
Weight (lb)	4'10"	4'11 "	5'0"	5'1"	5'2"	5'3"	5'4"	5'5"	5'6"	5'7"	5'8"	5'9"	5'10"	5'11"	6'0"	6'1"	6'2"
125	26	25	24	24	23	22	22	21	20	20	19	18	18	17	17	17	16
130	27	26	25	25	24	23	22	22	21	20	20	19	19	18	18	17	17
135	28	27	26	26	25	24	23	23	22	21	21	20	19	19	18	18	17
140	29	28	27	27	26	25	24	23	23	22	21	21	20	20	19	19	18
145	30	29	28	27	27	26	25	24	23	23	22	21	21	20	20	19	19
150	31	30	29	28	27	27	26	25	24	24	23	22	22	21	20	20	19
155	32	31	30	29	28	28	27	26	25	24	24	23	22	22	21	20	20
160	34	32	31	30	29	28	28	27	26	25	24	24	23	22	22	21	21
165	35	33	32	31	30	29	28	28	27	26	25	24	24	23	22	22	21
170	36	34	33	32	31	30	29	28	28	27	26	25	24	24	23	22	22
175	37	35	34	33	32	31	30	29	28	27	27	26	25	24	24	23	23
180	38	36	35	34	33	32	31	30	29	28	27	27	26	25	25	24	23
185	39	37	36	35	34	33	32	31	30	29	28	27	27	26	25	24	24
190	40	38	37	36	35	34	33	32	31	30	29	28	27	27	26	25	24
195	41	39	38	37	36	35	34	33	32	31	30	29	28	27	27	26	25
200	42	40	39	38	37	36	34	33	32	31	30	30	29	28	27	26	26
205	43	41	40	39	38	36	35	34	33	32	31	30	29	29	28	27	26
210	44	43	41	40	38	37	36	35	34	33	32	31	30	29	29	28	27
215	45	44	42	41	39	38	37	36	35	34	33	32	31	30	29	28	28
220	46	45	43	42	40	39	38	37	36	35	34	33	32	31	30	29	28
225	47	46	44	43	41	40	39	38	36	35	34	33	32	31	31	30	29
230	48	47	45	44	42	41	40	38	37	36	35	34	33	32	31	30	30
235	49	48	46	44	43	42	40	39	38	37	36	35	34	33	32	31	30
240	50	49	47	45	44	43	41	40	39	38	37	36	35	34	33	32	31
245	51	50	48	46	45	43	42	41	40	38	37	36	35	34	33	32	32
250	52	51	49	47	46	44	43	42	40	39	38	37	36	35	34	33	32
255	53	52	50	48	47	45	44	43	41	40	39	38	37	36	35	34	33
260	54	53	51	49	48	46	45	43	42	41	40	38	37	36	35	34	33
265	56	54	52	50	49	47	46	44	43	42	40	39	38	37	36	35	34
270	57	55	53	51	49	48	46	45	44	42	41	40	39	38	37	36	35
275	58	56	54	52	50	49	47	46	44	43	42	41	40	38	37	36	35
280	59	57	55	53	51	50	48	47	45	44	43	41	40	39	38	37	36
285	60	58	56	54	52	51	49	48	46	45	43	42	41	40	39	38	37
290	61	59	57	55	53	51	50	48	47	46	44	43	42	41	39	38	37
295	62	60	58	56	54	52	51	49	48	46	45	44	42	41	40	39	38
300	63	61	59	57	55	53	52	50	48	47	46	44	43	42	41	40	39
305	64	62	60	58	56	54	52	51	49	48	46	45	44	43	41	40	39
310	65	63	61	59	57	55	53	52	50	49	47	46	45	43	42	41	40
315	66	64	62	60	58	56	54	53	51	49	48	47	45	44	43	42	41
320	67	65	63	61	59	57	55	53	52	50	49	47	46	45	43	42	41
325	68	66	64	62	60	58	56	54	53	51	50	48	47	45	44	43	42

Antihistamines prevent the release of histamine. Histamine is the chemical released from certain cells in the body after being exposed to an allergen. It causes the swelling of the membranes in the nose and increases mucus production. During an allergic reaction, you will have symptoms such as a runny nose, itchy eyes, and nasal stuffiness.

Check out Table 7.4 to find medications that will work in your situation.

TABLE 7.4: ANTIHISTAMINES

Non-Sedating or Mildly Sedating	
Generic Name	**Brand Name**
Terfenadine	Seldane
Astemizole	Hismanal
Loratadine	Claritin
Cetirizine	Zyrtec
Fexofenadine	Allegra
Sedating	
Generic Name	Brand Name
Brompheniramine	Dimetane
Chlorpheniramine	Chlortrimeton
Diphenhydramine	Benadryl
Tripelennamine	PBZ
Promethazine	Phenergan
Azatadine	Optimine
Hydroxyzine	Atarax, Vistaril
Clemastine	Tavist
Cyproheptadine	Periactin

Sedating antihistamines may cause you other problems besides sleepiness. If you take these drugs, you may have decreased reaction time and a hard time paying attention. Other side effects include a dry mouth, overly dry nose, painful or difficult urination, urinary retention, blurred vision, and constipation.

Non-sedating antihistamines do not cause drowsiness or these other side effects, but terfenadine (Seldane) and astemizole (Hismanal) have been associated with abnormal heart rhythms. These two drugs need to be prescribed with particular caution and avoided in people who have liver disease, as well as other chronic medical problems. Some non-sedating antihistamines should never be taken at the same time as antifungal drugs (ketoconazole or itraconazole) or the antibiotic erythromycin. The other sedating antihistamines do not have these restrictions, and all are available in combination with a decongestant. Because decongestants may raise your blood pressure and heart rate, elderly people or those suffering from hypertension or heart conditions should avoid these.

Decongestants work by reducing blood flow to the turbinates (spongy bones within the nose), which helps to reduce the swelling. When you use a decongestant spray directly into your nose, it works rapidly and is more effective than if you take this as a pill. Don't take decongestant sprays for more than five to seven days because they can produce a "rebound effect." This means that the ongoing usage of the inhaled decongestant causes an irritation and/or an increase in the swelling of the turbinates. While this swelling wears off if the medication is stopped, it may produce a vicious cycle of overuse. In other words, the relief you feel will be short lived, which makes you use the spray more frequently. If you do use a spray decongestant, try the longer-acting form, and remember to observe the "short-term usage" rule.

Oral decongestants can cause side effects such as tremors, jitters, nervousness, difficulty falling asleep, and difficulty urinating, especially in men with enlarged prostate glands. The inhalant spray decongestants are less likely to cause side effects except the rebound effect. If overused they may produce nasal septum perforations. Again, if you have heart problems or high blood pressure, avoid decongestants altogether.

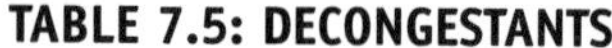

TABLE 7.5: DECONGESTANTS

Oral	
Generic Name	**Brand Name**
Pseudoephedrine	Sudafed, Novafed
Phenylpropanolamine	
Phenylephrine	
Inhalant long-acting (eight to 12 hours)	
Oxymetazoline	Afrin
Xylometazoline	Neosynephrine, 12-hr/maximum Sinex, Otrixin
Inhalant short-acting (three to eight hours)	
Tetrahydrozoline	
Naphazoline	Privine
Phenylephrine	Vicks, Duration, Neo-Synephrine

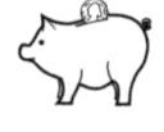

Moneysaver
Before you spend your money on a touted "snoring cure," it's important to know that the U.S. Patent Office has more than 300 would-be snoring remedies, but most are not helpful. Ask your doctor before you launch out on your own.

Other helpful medications include:

- Anticholinergics—a form of medication to treat nasal congestion that may help decrease your snoring. This type of medicine is helpful for those with a clear, watery discharge (rhinorrhea) from the nose. The most effective one available today is *ipratropium bromide* (Atrovent), an inhalant that comes in two strengths. {The 0.03 percent preparation is useful for allergic and non-allergic rhinitis when the clear, watery discharge is a prominent problem; the 0.06 percent strength is useful when the common cold (coryza) caused by a virus produces nasal drip.} The most common side effect is irritation or excessive nasal dryness that can lead to nose bleeds.

- Cromolyn sodium (Nasalcrom)—a type of medication that blocks the allergic response to allergens. It prevents mast cells, which are located in the linings of the nose, trachea, and bronchial tubes, from releasing histamine. Cromolyn sodium works if you use it *before* exposure and should be taken a week or so before the allergy season begins. The benefit of cromolyn sodium is that there are no side effects.
- Corticosteroids—the most effective medications available for the treatment of nasal congestion due to allergy or non-allergic causes. With steroids, the oral therapy is more effective and gets started more quickly than topical or inhaled usage. Topical treatment with cromolyn or inhaled steroids may follow this oral therapy. Again, steroids and cromolyn work over time—they must be taken *daily*.

There are now at least six topical or inhaled steroids available by prescription (see Table 7.6). Dexamethasone is the most potent, yet this drug may be absorbed in its active form and produce some serious side effects. The other drugs are less likely to be absorbed and are metabolized or cleared quickly from the blood stream if absorbed. They produce few if any side effects if taken in recommended doses. Nasal irritation is the most common side effect. Sometimes this is severe enough to produce nasal bleeding. If this happens, stop the medicine immediately. Perforation of the nasal septum can occur, and you need to be aware of this problem.

There are many types of containers for inhaled sprays. Work with your doctor to find the best one for your problem. Usually these sprays can be taken for several months without a problem, but some doctors recommend that they be used for only five to 14 days at a time. When your nasal congestion is relieved, you might stop the spray for a while before it is needed again for another period of treatment.

TABLE 7.6: NASAL STEROID INHALERS

Generic Name	Brand Name
Dexamethasone	Dexacort
Beclomethasone	Beconase, Vancenase
Budesonide	Rhinocort
Flunisolide	Nasalide, Nasarel
Fluticasone	Flonase
Triamcinolone	Nasacort
Mometasone	Nasonex

For some people with nasal congestion due to allergies, taking control of your environment may make a big difference. In some cases, eliminating environmental triggers may even cure your snoring problem.

Go through your home or office, and discover the problem areas. Environmental triggers vary. See Table 7.7 for a list of common triggers.

TABLE 7.7: COMMON ENVIRONMENTAL TRIGGERS

Aerosols	Chemical fumes
Cigarette smoke	Cockroaches (feces)
Cold air	Dust
Fresh paint	Humid air
Mold and mildew	Perfume
Pet dander	Pollen
Scented products	Tobacco and wood smoke
Weather fronts	Wind

Try nasal dilators

Various nasal dilators have been tried for years to help relieve the obstruction inside the nose. Some of these devices are inserted into the nostrils. Needless to say, these have not been popular because of their discomfort and the high level of maintenance required to keep them clean. An external dilator called "Breathe Right Nasal Strips" has been marketed with some success. These strips are available at most drug and grocery stores and are worn on the outside of the nose. They are designed to slightly open the nose near the tip. When stuck to the skin on the front of your nose, the Breathe Right Nasal Strip stabilizes the outer walls of the nasal passages with a springboard action to prevent collapse during inhalation. An increased outer opening of your nose tends to decrease resistance to airflow, which may also result in less mouth breathing.

If your snoring is mainly due to narrowing of the nasal passages, these strips may reduce or eliminate the snoring. Be patient when using these, as it may take a week or two to get back into the habit of keeping your mouth closed while asleep. Also keep in mind that snoring and airway obstruction during apneas occur behind the soft palate and tongue. In these cases, nasal dilators probably will not be helpful in treating sleep apnea. If you are using positive airway pressure therapy, these nasal strips may be helpful in preventing nasal obstruction.

Other commonly used "cures" for snoring include:

- A change of sleep position, type of pillow, and elevating head of bed. Often simply sleeping on your side instead of your back or changing from a feather pillow to a foam pillow can put a stop to your snoring cycle.

- Dental appliances—a wide range of devices that fit into the mouth during sleep. Some devices can reduce snoring in about three-quarters of the people who wear them regularly.
- Alternative treatments—natural enzymes that break up the mucus in the throat; root, herb, and flower extracts that open the sinuses and contract the uvula, among others.
- Various devices designed to pull the tongue forward have been used, as well as devices that pull the jawbone forward. While these devices work, they may be uncomfortable and reduce the quality of your sleep.
- Tracheostomy, which was the gold-standard for treating OSA 20 years ago. Today, however, acceptance of this method is low because of cosmetic reasons and complications such as bleeding or infection. Occasionally this treatment is still used in emergency situations.

Medications that help to improve upper airway muscle strength or tone during sleep, as well as help to increase REM sleep, are also available. If you have an underactive thyroid (hypothyroidism), thyroid hormone replacement is clearly useful. Antidepressant drugs have worked well in some with mild OSA. These agents decrease the amount of REM sleep, the sleep stage during which apneas tend to be more severe, thus improving the sleep-related breathing disorder indirectly. These drugs also may work by stimulating nerves that control muscles responsible for keeping your upper airway open.

Protriptyline, which is non-sedating, is one of the best-studied antidepressants used for sleep apnea. It is used in a dose of 5 mg to 20 mg at bedtime. The drawbacks are the annoying side effects that increase as the dosage is raised. These include dry mouth, urinary hesitancy and/or frequency, and impotence. Another antidepressant, fluoxetine (Prozac), is also helpful to reduce the respiratory disturbance index. Side effects of this drug, however, may be lower libido, loss of appetite or nausea. If you have sleep apnea, be careful to avoid alcohol and drugs such as benzodiazepines (Xanax, Valium, and Restoril), which depress the central nervous system, relax the upper airway musculature, and may worsen sleep apnea.

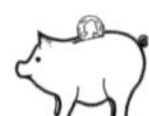

Moneysaver
If you snore and are overweight, losing 10 pounds could stop your snoring and also save you money on unnecessary tests and treatment.

CPAP, the Treatment of Choice for OSA

Nasal continuous positive airway pressure (nasal CPAP) is now the treatment of choice for OSA. *It is almost 100 percent effective and safe for stopping snoring and OSA.* While CPAP is not invasive, it eliminates snoring and reduces the number of sleep-related breathing problems. By doing so, it decreases fragmented sleep and results in fewer problems of daytime sleepiness, fatigue, and mood and memory problems.

CPAP works by maintaining a positive pressure inside your airway while you breathe. It acts as a support to prevent further narrowing or collapse of your airway, and it actually increases the size of the airway behind the palate and at the back of your tongue.

CPAP is usually applied by a custom-made, custom-fit mask that is strapped onto your nose. This mask is connected by a swivel and flexible hose to a special pump that quietly provides air under pressure to your nose. Instead of the nasal mask, you may prefer "nasal pillows," which are inserted into your nostrils. In some cases, a chinstrap is helpful to keep your mouth closed to reduce loss of pressure. A full-face mask may be necessary in select cases.

While you are asleep in a sleep-disorders laboratory, the doctor will be able to find the optimal CPAP level you need to get rid of snoring and the other episodes of narrowing in the upper airway.

The first sleep study diagnoses OSA and determines its nature and severity. If nasal CPAP is determined by your doctor to be the best treatment, a second study will be necessary. During the second sleep study, the pressure is then adjusted to the lowest amount needed to relieve the decreases in airflow and to maximize the oxygen levels in your blood during sleep. In some cases, a split-night polysomnogram may be necessary. This involves being monitored for sleep-related breathing abnormalities the first part of the night. If significant sleep apnea is found, then during the second part of the night, you will try nasal CPAP to find the right pressure necessary to end symptoms of OSA.

During daytime hours at the sleep clinic, you will be introduced to the mask and machine. You will try it on and see what it's like breathing with the CPAP machine. If you find it reasonably comfortable and your nose has a good flow of air, then another night in the sleep laboratory is scheduled. On the second night in the laboratory, all the sleep stage parameters and respiratory factors, including airflow and oxygen levels, are monitored again. If you understand this process ahead of time, this second night is much more successful. After the required level of CPAP is determined, your doctor will arrange to have the proper mask and machine, which is set at the appropriate pressure, delivered to your home.

CPAP is not, however, perfect. Some of the common problems many find with CPAP include:

- Psychological aversion
- Claustrophobia
- Arousals from sleep
- Nasal discomfort, especially dryness
- Swallowing air and stomach cramps
- Leaks at nose or mouth
- Facial skin irritation
- Discomfort exhaling
- Chest or back pain

Bright Idea
If your bed partner sleeps in another room at night or lies awake as a passive listener to your snoring, ending these nocturnal sounds will allow both of you to get the healing rest you need and awaken feeling refreshed.

Curing Snoring and OSA with Surgery

You've tried the non-surgical treatments, yet are still unable to cure snoring. Don't worry, you are not alone. There are more steps in finding the snoring cure for your specific situation. While the final step in curing snoring is a bit more drastic—*it does work in most cases.* This is when you must eliminate what is aggravating those noisy Zzzz.

The best surgical alternatives recommended to cure snoring include:

- Tonsillectomy and/or adenoidectomy—tonsils and adenoids are collections of lymph tissue found in the airways. If these are swollen, they can obstruct normal breathing and cause snoring. An ear, nose, and throat surgeon performs this surgery in an operating room.
- Uvulopalatopharyngoplasty (UPPP)—performed by an ear/nose/throat surgeon in the operating room with a scalpel (see Figure 7.2). This proce-

dure has a success rate of about *50 to 90 percent* and involves removal of tonsils and adenoids, if present, and excision of the uvula and most of the soft palate, resulting in a larger pharyngeal airway at the end of the soft palate. The cost for this surgery is approximately $10,000 to $12,000, and it requires general anesthesia and a long recovery.

- Laser-assisted uvulopalatoplasty (LAUP)—a 15- to 30-minute office procedure to trim and reshape the uvula and soft palate, requiring only a local anesthetic (see Figure 7.3). It has a success rate of curing snoring of about 95 percent. It may require three to five visits—with one month of healing time in between—and cost around $1,500 to $2,000 in most parts of the nation. During the office procedure, you remain upright and awake, and leave with *no* stitches and only a minor sore throat. Those who have had laser surgery say it could be compared to the "amount of time and stress experienced with having a cavity filled."
- Nasal polypectomy, nasal septoplasty, or other surgeries to correct abnormalities that cause obstruction to airflow in the nose. These operating-room surgeries help to correct a deviated nasal septum. This is where the partition that separates the two nasal cavities is curved or not aligned. Some people have polyps or growths in their nose that hinder breathing and make it chronically stuffy. Removal of polyps may cure their snoring.
- Tracheostomy—although this bypasses airway obstruction and has generally been replaced by

CPAP, tracheostomy is still reserved for the most critically ill persons, such as those with life-threatening cardiac dysrhythmias. It is effective in virtually all persons and can be used temporarily while a person loses weight for reversal of OSA.

- Weight reduction surgery done in the operating room by a surgeon, involving shrinking the size of the stomach or through bypassing the stomach, which may solve the problem for the obese snorer. As with all types of surgery, the risks must be weighed with the benefits.

FIGURE 7.2: UVULOPALATOPHARYNGOPLASTY (UPPP)

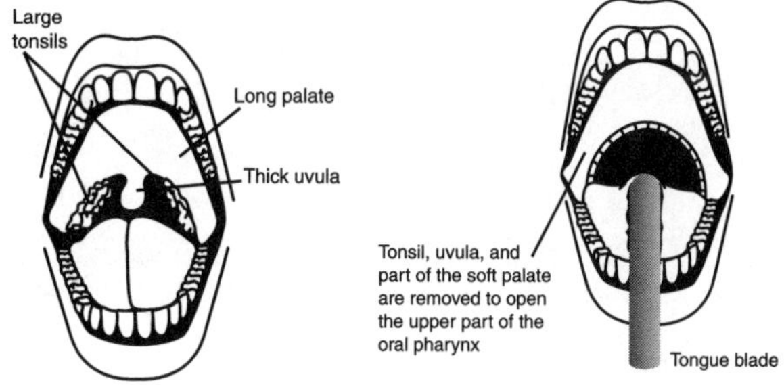

FIGURE 7.3: LASER-ASSISTED UVULOPALATOPLASTY (LAUP)

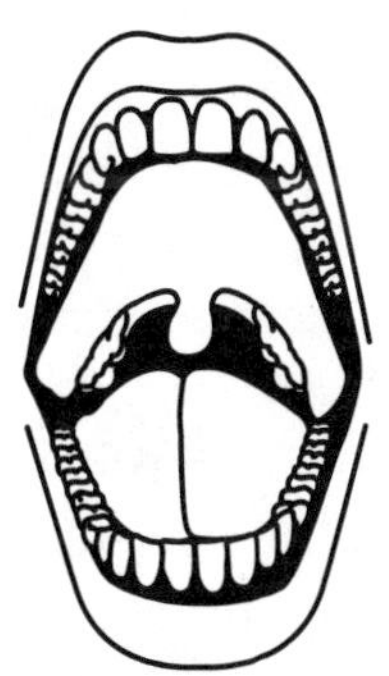

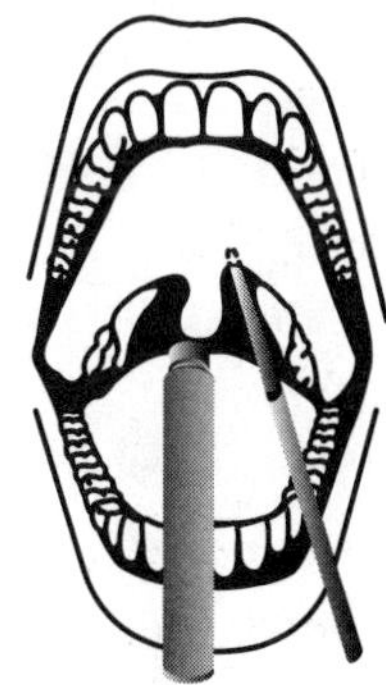

The Benefits of Treatment

Treatment for snoring really does work. Researchers have found that successfully curing snoring and OSA will also do the following:

Boost your immune function

Snoring is guaranteed to disrupt your sleep cycle, resulting in less REM (Rapid Eye Movement) sleep. It is during Stage 4, the deepest level of sleep, that the body is revitalized and tissue damage is repaired. In fact, a lack of deep sleep is associated with reduced immune function. Taking care of the snoring will enable you to sleep sounder through the night, greatly enhancing your body's ability to resist diseases and infections.

Lower your blood pressure

More than one-third of those with hypertension also have OSA. The majority of those with severe sleep apnea are hypertensive. Uncontrolled hypertension can lead to serious cardiovascular problems, including increased risk of angina and heart disease (see Chapter 5). Fortunately, hypertension often improves after treatment of OSA.

Improved cardiovascular function

If you snore and have OSA, chances are your heart is being greatly stressed. Studies show that habitual snorers (as compared to non-snorers) have a greater chance of stroke, and an increased chance that the stroke will be fatal. It is not unusual for those with sleep apnea to be mistakenly treated for primary heart disease because cardiac arrhythmias may be more prominent than the breathing disturbances.

When breathing stops during the apneas, your heart rate and level of oxygen also drop, you pump less blood out, and your blood pressure increases.

When breathing resumes, your heart rate and blood pressure rise, sometimes to very dangerous levels. These problems are lessened when treatment begins to correct the snoring and OSA.

Increased sex drive

It has long been suspected that hypertension and erectile dysfunction are associated. Some medications for hypertension and other medical problems can also cause male sexual dysfunction. Because male impotence is directly related to OSA, taking care of the OSA can often help solve associated sexual problems, including erectile dysfunction. For the "pure" or asymptomatic snorer, ending this annoying noise will allow your bed partner to move back into your bed and sleep with you once again.

> "You probably know what it's like to get a bad night's sleep. But what if you were married to someone who snored and has not slept soundly in years? Snoring has virtually ruined our marriage.
> —Thelma, homemaker, 53"

Greater energy, alertness, and productivity

Sleep deprivation caused by snoring and OSA can make you feel moody, tired, and mentally impaired. In fact, researchers claim that those with OSA have more car accidents and sick days than non-snorers. People with OSA also have poor concentration, impaired memory, and do poorly on psychological testing. The low levels of oxygen in the blood may be the cause of this problem; correcting it may let you experience all stages of sleep and rejuvenate your body.

Getting Some *Zzzzs*

There are many options available that can help you enjoy healing and restful sleep, as well as solve the impotence associated with OSA. Talk with your doctor or sleep disorders specialist about specific concerns, and seek appropriate medication or treatment.

Just the Facts

- Snoring can be a symptom of OSA, as can impotence.
- OSA differs from "pure" snoring, but consult your doctor if you suffer from any sleep disorder.
- Diagnosis and treatment can end snoring that is annoying for your partner and potentially life-threatening for you.
- A wide variety of treatments are available.
- Treatment offers collateral benefits such as lower blood pressure and increased sex drive.

Chapter 8

GET THE SCOOP ON...
Baby boomers and osteoarthritis ▪ Free and easy pain relief for arthritis ▪ American men and fractures from osteoporosis ▪ Male risk factors for osteoporosis

The Problems of Arthritis and Osteoporosis

If you suffer with arthritis or osteoporosis, even the thought of having sex may make you run. Why? Think about enjoying the act of making love when your joints are stiff and aching or your muscles throb with each movement. Every time you turn over on your side or back, you feel intense stabbing or penetrating pain in the hips or back. Or if you have osteoporosis (thin bones), getting into a comfortable position associated with making love may be impossible due to back pain from a fracture or the results of deformity. In fact, in some people with osteoporosis, movement during sex could be enough to cause a fracture.

This constant, chronic pain may easily be a direct factor in your impotence. Chronic pain causes fatigue, depression, less activity, and commonly decreases libido. When joint pain, especially in the hips, knees, or back, becomes worse during sexual activity, then further erection problems may follow. The fear of failure may complicate and compound the problems with sexual function.

If you have arthritis, there is no reason you can't still enjoy an active sex life. It's important to control the pain and stiffness as much as possible with moist heat, exercises, and medications, as outlined in this chapter.

For those with osteoporosis, keeping your bones strong by eating a diet high in calcium and vitamin D, as well as enjoying regular weight-bearing exercise and taking new medications, may also allow you to enjoy sex without fear of injury.

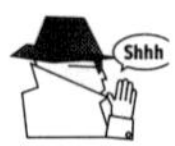

Unofficially... There are over 100 types of arthritis, and over 40 million Americans are affected.

In both cases, if erectile dysfunction is a problem, discuss it with your doctor or rheumatologist (arthritis specialist), who can ensure there are no other contributing causes that could be eliminated with treatment.

There are solutions to problems with arthritis and osteoporosis. But before we present the best treatments—which do not have impotence as a side effect—it's important to understand these two common conditions associated with aging.

Arthritis Leads to Unending Pain

Arthritis means inflammation in or around the joints. This causes pain, swelling, and stiffness in the hands, wrists, elbows, shoulders, hips, knees, ankles, feet, neck, or back. The pain and stiffness can begin suddenly or may appear over years.

TABLE 8.1: TWO MAIN GROUPS OF ARTHRITIS

Inflammatory Arthritis	Osteoarthritis
Rheumatoid Arthritis	Fibromyalgia
Ankylosing Spondylitis	Bursitis
Systemic Lupus Erythematosus (SLE)	Tendinitis
Gout (Gouty Arthritis)	
Pseudogout	
PMR (Polymyalgia Rheumatica)	
Others	

The baby boomer's disease

The most common type of arthritis is osteoarthritis, in which the cartilage becomes worn and less efficient in cushioning the joints. Studies show that millions of baby boomers are in line for osteoarthritis as it is associated with increased age. After age 50, an estimated 80 percent of America's population is affected with osteoarthritis to some degree and may have signs of pain and stiffness. Some studies show that almost everyone over the age of 60 has some form of osteoarthritis, although not all will have the symptoms (see Figure 8.1).

With America's rapidly aging population, by the year 2010, when the first wave of baby boomers hit their mid-sixties, it is predicted that there will be more than 70 million people with osteoarthritis. That's a lot of aching joints!

Check the list of common risk factors for osteoarthritis in Table 8.2 to see if you are at risk. If you are, try to change any you can control. For example, obesity is a risk factor for osteoarthritis, so losing weight would be one positive step you could take to reduce this risk.

FIGURE 8.1: OSTEOARTHRITIC HAND

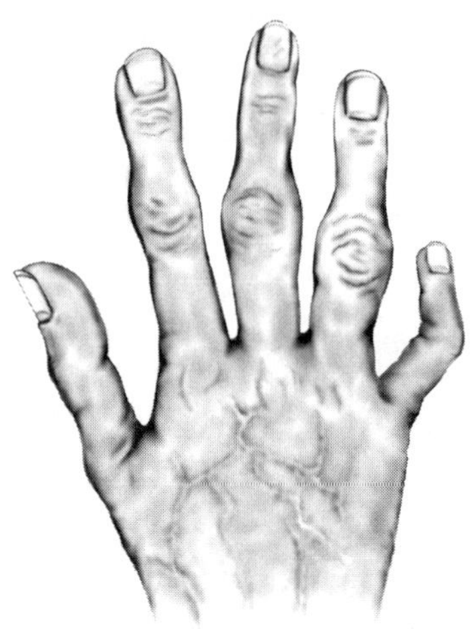

> "I played football for almost a decade. Now I can hardly put weight on my feet because of osteoarthritis in my ankles.
> —Sam, insurance salesman, 38"

TABLE 8.2: COMMON RISK FACTORS FOR OSTEOARTHRITIS

Increased age	Injury
Athletes	Heavy, constant joint use
Knee surgery	Abnormal joint positions
Gender	Changing forces or positions of joints
Obesity	Lack of exercise
Joint injury by other types of arthritis	

Osteoarthritis—the "wear and tear" arthritis—is the most common type of arthritis. While age is a big factor in who gets osteoarthritis, that's not always the case. For example, many young women in their early twenties and thirties suffer from osteoarthritis in the hands, and young athletes or dancers can have arthritis in their knees, ankles, hips, or other joints stemming from injuries.

Osteoarthritis can affect almost any joint, but is most typical in the joints that bear weight over the years, such as the knees, hips, and lower back. The pain and stiffness usually come on gradually over months or even years. But in many cases, the joints primarily affected are those that allow us to lead active lives, such as the back, hips, and knees we depend on for walking; the back, shoulders, and hands for lifting; or the back, hips, knees, and hands for working.

Your doctor makes the diagnosis after discussion and examination and usually confirms it with x-rays, which show loss or wearing of the cartilage and spur formation around the joint. If fluid is removed from the joint, tests on the fluid can confirm the diagnosis and may give temporary relief of the joint pain and stiffness.

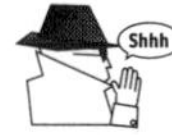

Unofficially... Arthritis causes up to $17 billion in lost earnings in people under the age of 65—earning losses of 25 to 50 percent compared to those with no arthritis.

Rheumatoid arthritis has an unknown cause

The next most common types of arthritis are those in which the lining of the joints becomes inflamed. The most common type is rheumatoid arthritis, although there are many types of arthritis that may look like rheumatoid arthritis. The cause is unknown, but it brings pain and swelling in the hands, wrists, elbows, shoulders, knees, ankles, feet, and hips in some combination. There is usually stiffness in the morning upon awakening, which may take hours to disappear. And there is often fatigue, which can be severe and limiting.

Rheumatoid arthritis can affect almost any age, but is actually most common between the ages of 20 and 40 and 50 and 60. It is more common in women but happens in men as well.

FMS leaves you too tired for sex

Fibromyalgia Syndrome (FMS) is an arthritis-like syndrome that can make you dread sexual intercourse because of constant deep muscle pain and fatigue, similar to that with the flu. Fibromyalgia is usually diagnosed in females, ages 20 to 55, but if you have the symptoms, better get it checked out. Although fibromyalgia commonly affects more women than men, it does occur in men.

Fibromyalgia is a common cause of deep muscle pain in the arms, legs, neck, shoulders, and back. It can look and feel similar to osteoarthritis, bursitis, and tendinitis, and sometimes it is misdiagnosed as chronic fatigue syndrome (CFS).

Although the cause is unknown, some researchers think fibromyalgia may result from a genetic tendency that is passed on from generation to generation. When a person who has this tendency is exposed to certain emotional or physical stressors (like in an illness), there is a change in their body's response to stress. This can result in a higher sensitivity of the entire body to pain. Scientists theorize that one of these body changes is a low level of the hormone CRH (corticotropin-releasing hormone), resulting in higher sensitivity to pain and more fatigue, including the fatigue experienced after exercise.

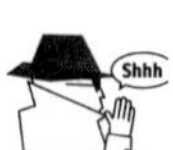

Unofficially... Studies show that women have a 10-times greater chance of getting fibromyalgia than men, and figures tell of fibromyalgia affecting more than 10 million people in America today.

This hypersensitivity to pain may in part be from low levels of serotonin. Serotonin is a neurotransmitter in the brain associated with a calming, anxiety-reducing reaction. Lower levels of serotonin cause a lower pain threshold. The end result may be the chronic widespread pain of fibromyalgia.

Still other researchers have recently concluded that those with fibromyalgia have significantly less blood flow to the parts of the brain that deal with pain. In studies where fibromyalgia patients were compared to healthy people, those with fibromyalgia were found to have twice the level of a brain chemical called Substance P, a neuropeptide involved in pain signals. This chemical helps nervous system cells send messages to each other about painful stimuli. It is thought that when Substance P levels are elevated in the body, they may produce higher levels of pain.

The term fibromyalgia or fibrositis implies that there is inflammation of fibrous tissue in the muscles and other tissues, but this has not been proven when samples of those tissues were studied.

In fibromyalgia, the areas most commonly affected are the neck, shoulders, elbows, knees, and back. Although there may be difficulty doing daily work or caring for the home, most people with this disease can complete these duties despite not feeling well. The symptoms and feelings usually come and go and commonly are associated with severe fatigue, headache, and depression. Most people have difficulty sleeping. They may be unable to get to sleep or may not feel rested when they awaken in the morning. On arising, they may feel stiffness in the muscles and joints. See the list of common symptoms of fibromyalgia in Table 8.3 to see if it might be affecting you.

“I went to four different doctors over a period of three years before one doctor finally diagnosed me with fibromyalgia syndrome. The other three doctors inferred that my symptoms were imagined or in my head.
—Alan, high school teacher, 36”

TABLE 8.3: COMMON SYMPTOMS OF FIBROMYALGIA

Pain	Morning stiffness	Localized muscle tenderness
Difficult or unrefreshing sleep	Anxiety	Lack of concentration
Depression	Swelling, numbness and tingling in hands, arms, feet, and legs	Headaches
Fatigue	Constipation, diarrhea, abdominal pain	Burning or frequent urination
Restless legs syndrome	Dryness in mouth, nose, and eyes	Discoloration of hands and feet (Raynaud's phenomenon)

The feelings of pain and stiffness in fibromyalgia are very widespread, unlike the osteoarthritis, bursitis, or tendinitis in which pain is localized to a single area. In fact, if there are not many areas involved, then it does not fit the typical picture of fibromyalgia.

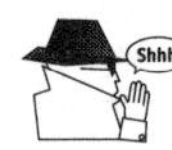

Unofficially... Gout, a common form of inflammatory arthritis, affects more than one million people, mostly men over age 40.

With fibromyalgia, there is no joint swelling, no loss of movement of the joints, and no true muscle weakness as one might experience with other problems. Usually the only abnormal findings are the tender areas over the neck, shoulder blades, lower back, elbows, and knees. These tender points are called trigger areas and can cause pain that is felt in other areas. In fact, if a joint is warm or swollen or does not move properly, there is probably another problem present (see Figure 8.2).

Fibromyalgia can happen alone or along with another problem such as rheumatoid arthritis, systemic lupus erythematosus (SLE or lupus), polymyalgia rheumatica, or other internal organ diseases.

Arthritis in men

Gout most commonly attacks the large toe with very severe pain, swelling, and redness in the joint. The pain is often too severe to walk or stand and may be so severe that even the weight of a bed sheet hurts the toe. It can also attack the ankle, knee, elbow, or other joints. More than one joint can be painful and swollen at times. The attacks usually go away in a few weeks, but if untreated, gout can return and cause a severe arthritis with deformity.

The cause of gout is a high blood level of uric acid, which crystalizes in the joints. After proper diagnosis, treatment is available to lower the uric acid level, which will prevent future attacks of gout.

Ankylosing spondylitis is yet another type of inflammatory arthritis that is most common in men, especially young men, and causes the joints of the lower back to become painful and stiff. This type of spinal arthritis affects more than 300,000 people and usually starts gradually as pain in the lower back that may come and go at first. Instead of improving as would be expected from a strain, it gradually worsens.

There is almost always morning stiffness that may last for hours. The pain and stiffness usually get worse with prolonged inactivity. Most persons do best if they keep some level of activity instead of staying sedentary. Half of those affected have arthritis in the shoulders or hips.

The pain often gradually moves from the lower back to the middle and upper back. After five to 10 years, the neck may also be affected. The spine may become so stiff that movement is very limited in any direction. This can make it difficult to bend, stoop, or even turn the head to drive a car. (The disease often finally "burns out" after years, and the pain can actually stop.)

Watch Out!
Gout can begin after another illness, surgery, or heavy alcohol intake, such as during a party weekend.

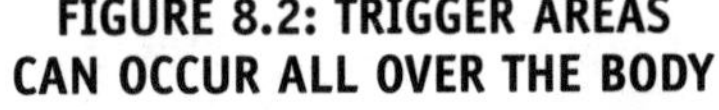

FIGURE 8.2: TRIGGER AREAS CAN OCCUR ALL OVER THE BODY

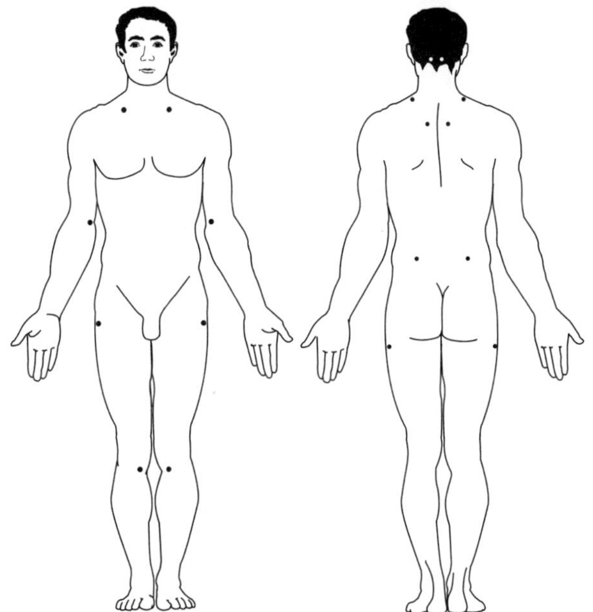

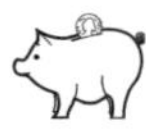

Moneysaver
Moist heat is the most effective form of treatment for minor aches and pains—and it's virtually free. Take advantage of a warm shower or bath twice a day after a weekend of exercise and activity.

The cause is not known, but treatment is available to control the pain and help prevent the possibility of severe deformity. If the spine becomes stiff in a straight, useful position, disability can be prevented.

Still hurting all over?

Other kinds of arthritis and related diseases are also thought to be due to wear-and-tear changes and are treated in ways similar to osteoarthritis. These include bursitis and tendinitis. Bursitis is due to inflammation in a bursa, which is a sac near a joint that allows the muscles and tendons to move more smoothly over the bones and joints. Bursitis is common around the shoulder, hip, and knee.

Tendinitis is due to inflammation around a tendon, which attaches a muscle to a bone. When the tendon is used, there is pain where the tendon attaches to the bone. This is common in the elbow (tennis elbow and golfer's elbow) and at the shoulder. Both tendinitis and bursitis are treated similarly to osteoarthritis.

Finding Effective Treatments

Treatment for both types of arthritis includes moist heat for the joints (like a warm shower or bath), medications to help relieve inflammation, and exercises to keep the joints limber and make the muscles stronger.

Moist heat is most effective

The first step in treatment of arthritis is simple and inexpensive—moist heat. For treatment of arthritis, moist heat offers many benefits because it:

- Relieves pain
- Relaxes tight muscles
- Loosens stiff joints
- Increases flexibility.

Moist heat makes it easier to exercise the arthritic joints and can allow movement of stiff joints to increase. Joint exercises are also easier and more effective with moist heat. Some of the best types of moist heat are listed in Table 8.4. See which type works best for your form of arthritis.

No matter which form of moist heat you use, be sure to do this application twice every day, without fail. Start with 15 minutes each morning and evening. If necessary, you might have to get up a few minutes earlier in the morning before your day starts, then repeat the treatment before bedtime. Your commitment of time and effort will be definitely worth the improvement you will feel. With the moist heat, you should feel some improvement in pain and stiffness almost immediately.

TABLE 8.4: COMMON TYPES OF MOIST HEAT

Warm shower (sit on chair, if needed)	Warm, moist towel or cloth	Warm bath
Warm whirlpool or hot tub	Heated swimming pool	Hot pack, such as a hydrocollator pack
Moist heating pad	Paraffin-mineral oil therapeutic mixture	

Medications alleviate pain and stiffness

The specific medications taken for arthritis do not usually cause erection problems, although you may disagree, depending on your personal experience.

There are two groups of medicines that are most effective for the pain. One is the group of medicines used to treat pain—the analgesics (see Table 8.5). The second group of medications used for treatment is the non-steroidal anti-inflammatory drugs (NSAIDs), listed in Table 8.6.

Bright Idea
If you experience stomach problems from arthritis medications, consider stopping the medications and taking one of the following over-the-counter preparations that actually block stomach acid production:

Axid
Pepcid
Tagamet
Zantac

Ask your doctor about antacids, medications that neutralize the acid after it is produced in the stomach, for prevention of ulcers and other problems caused by excess acid. Many different types are available over the counter.

Watch Out! You may be at higher risk for irritation or ulcers of the lining of the stomach when you take an NSAID if one of the following applies:

- If you had a stomach ulcer in the past.
- If you take a cortisone-type medication.
- If you smoke cigarettes.
- If you are over 65 years old.

If you have any unusual indigestion, heartburn, or abdominal pain, or if you notice any new problems, stop the medicine until you talk to your doctor.

TABLE 8.5: COMMONLY USED OVER-THE-COUNTER ANALGESICS TO RELIEVE PAIN

Trade Name	Generic Name
Advil	Ibuprofen
Aleve	Naproxyn sodium
Ascriptin (with Maalox)	Aspirin
Ecotrin, others	Enteric coated aspirin
8-Hour Bayer, Time Release	Aspirin
Many generic and store brands	Aspirin
Tylenol, Anacin-3, generic and store brands	Acetaminophen

TABLE 8.6: COMMONLY USED NON-STEROIDAL ANTI-INFLAMMATORY DRUGS

Trade Name	Generic Name	Trade Name	Generic Name
Advil	Ibuprofen	Anaprox	Naproxen
Ansaid	Flurbiprofen	Arthrotec	Diclofense plus Misoprostol
Clinoril	Sulindac	Daypro	Oxaprozin
Disalcid, Salflex, Monogesic	Salsalate	Dolobid	Diflunisal
Feldene	Piroxicam	Indocin	Indomethacin
Lodine	Etodolac	Magan	Magnesium salicylate
Meclomen	Meclofenamate	Nalfon	Fenoprofen
Naprosyn	Naproxen	Orudis	Ketoprofen
Oruvail	Ketoprofen delayed-release	Relafen	Nabumetone
Rufen	Ibuprofen	Tolectin	Tolmetin
Trilisate	Choline magnesium trisalicylate	Voltaren	Diclofenac
Zorprin	12-hour release aspirin		

Unwanted side effects

Even though most people do not experience side effects with these medications, it is important to always be on the lookout for any unwanted effects, especially if impotence is a concern. Then the medication can be stopped and the side effects minimized. The most common side effects (see Table 8.7) from arthritis medications are nausea, indigestion, heartburn, and upset stomach. Ulcers in the stomach (peptic ulcer disease) and intestine, intestinal bleeding, and abnormalities of the liver and kidney may also occur.

Cytotec (misoprostol) is a medication that protects the stomach lining before an anti-inflammatory drug can damage it. When taken along with one of the anti-inflammatory drugs, the risk of peptic ulcer disease and bleeding from the stomach or intestine is much lower.

Bright Idea
The National Osteoporosis Foundation in Washington, D.C., has prepared individualized "Bone Wise" kits for men of all ages. The men's kit contains four brochures about different aspects of osteoporosis as it applies to men, as well as information about preventing this debilitating disease. To get a free kit, call toll-free (888) 442-WISE (442-9473).

TABLE 8.7: COMMON SIDE EFFECTS OF NSAIDs

Indigestion	Heartburn	Abdominal pain
Gastritis	Peptic ulcer	Intestinal bleeding
Diarrhea	Constipation	Lower hemoglobin (anemia)
Itching	Palpitations	Sodium retention with edema (swelling)
Dizziness	Rash	Increased blood pressure (hypertension)
Headaches	Sleepiness	Abnormal liver tests (blood tests)
Confusion (especially in older patients)	Mouth ulcers	Asthma in those allergic
Ringing in the ears (tinnitus)	Depression	Fatigue
Occasional blurred vision	Difficulty sleeping	Sun sensitivity
Lowered white cells in blood count	Diminished effect of diuretics	May affect other medications taken
Meningitis-like illness (rare)	Can aggravate or cause kidney (renal) failure	
May decrease platelet effect (can affect bleeding)	May change the effect of other medication	Other individual allergic or unusual reactions

> "Most of my patients with all degrees of severity of arthritis who maintain a regular exercise program are able to see and feel improvement and prevent further pain and disability. Likewise, it is those people who do not use exercise as part of their daily routine who usually experience much less relief from the painful symptoms.
> —Caroline, rheumatologist, 57"

Avoiding impotence

As with any medication, when you take drugs for arthritis, be sure to follow the directions and the dosage listed on the container, unless your doctor directs otherwise. Medications differ in the intervals between doses, and each has important precautions that help to make them safe to use. If you are taking any other medications, check with your doctor before you begin taking a pain medication to be sure that combining drugs won't create a problem.

When cortisone-type medications are taken orally (but not by injection into the joint), some patients find problems with erection, although researchers have yet to determine if the erectile dysfunction is from the severe pain of the arthritis or from the medication itself.

If your doctor approves, a trial of Viagra for erectile dysfunction may improve your erections. If you continue to have erection problems, see a urologist and check out the other treatments discussed in this book.

Exercise decreases pain and increases sexual prowess

The three different types of exercise that will help you include:

- Range-of-motion or stretching exercises. These involve moving a joint as far as it will go (without pain) or through its full range-of-motion.
- Endurance or conditioning exercises. These involve cardiovascular forms of exercise such as walking, running, biking, swimming, rowing, or aerobics.
- Strengthening exercises. These exercises help to build strong muscles, ligaments, and tendons needed to support your body.

The following exercises and activities in Table 8.8 can often be easily incorporated into most prevention and treatment programs for osteoarthritis. Ask your doctor if one of these may help your situation.

TABLE 8.8: ACTIVITIES AND EXERCISES TO KEEP YOU STRONG AND FLEXIBLE

Badminton	Baseball	Basketball	Biking
Bowling	Dancing	Gardening	Golf
Handball	High-impact aerobics	Hiking	House cleaning
Karate	Kick boxing	Jumping rope	Low-impact aerobics
Mall walking	Mowing the lawn	In-line skating	Rollerskating
Rowing	Running	Soccer	Softball
Stair-climbing	Stationary cycling	Strength training	Swimming
Tai Chi	Tae kwon do	Tennis	Vacuuming
Walking	Washing windows	Water exercises	Yoga

Osteoporosis and Men

Men may think that osteoporosis, or thinning of the bones, is a woman's disease, but keep reading. This bone-wasting disease occurs slowly and silently and has been tagged "a woman's disease" because women are far more vulnerable to it and the fractures it causes. Half of all women develop it, and one woman in two over the age of 65 suffers one or more bone fractures because of it. But don't turn the page yet. Men do get osteoporosis!

Are you at risk?

One and a half million men in this country already have osteoporosis, and 3.5 million more are at high risk of developing it. The most common risk factor is age. Bones in men and women continue to become denser until about the age of 30, then gradually thin out.

Timesaver
No time to work out? Exercise throughout your day. Park your car at the end of the parking lot at work, take the stairs instead of the elevator, walk your dog, play with your children, and do your own housework. All of these exercises and activities will increase your aerobic strength and help keep muscles and joints strong.

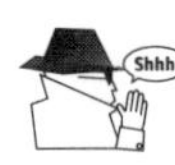

Unofficially... More than 20 percent of American men will suffer at least one fracture because their bones have become too thin and weak to withstand the normal stresses of life.

Though bone may seem solid and immutable, it is a tissue in constant flux. Calcium and other minerals are continually being leached from bone and replaced by minerals in the blood that are absorbed through the gut from foods and supplements. If the amount of restorative minerals falls short of what is lost or if the hormones that influence bone density are in short supply, the bones slowly get weaker.

In women, particularly those who do not take replacement estrogen, bone loss accelerates dramatically within the first five years or so after the onset of menopause. Since women usually start out with thinner bones than do men, this loss puts them at great risk of fractures as they age. Men do not experience a sudden dramatic decline in bone mass, but their more gradual losses add up. The older a man is, the greater his bone loss is likely to be, in part, because testosterone gradually decreases with age. Testosterone is crucial to bone strength in men, just as estrogen is crucial in women.

Nonetheless, as one 52-year-old man learned the hard way, you do not have to be "old" to develop osteoporosis. In an interview conducted by the National Osteoporosis Foundation, the man, a golfer, said his first indication of a problem had been an intense pain in his back as he swung his club. The diagnosis: an osteoporotic fracture of a vertebra. Another man, a 53-year-old, was forced by fragile bones to take early retirement from a job he loved.

Falls lead to fractures

A simple fall that in boyhood resulted in a scraped elbow or knee can mean a fractured wrist or hip for an older man. And hip fractures are serious; one-third of men with hip fractures die within a year from complications of the fracture or its treatment. Because grown men rarely have their height checked, many are unaware of the inches they lose with age, the consequence of vertebral fractures caused by osteoporosis.

Somctimes these spinal fractures are all too apparent, causing severe back pain and a bent posture. Nonetheless, many men wait for the discomfort to subside and ignore the developing spinal deformity. However, osteoporosis in men and women can nearly always be prevented. If the condition is detected early, treatment can prevent significant bone loss and fractures.

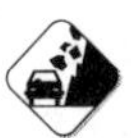

Watch Out!
Men are especially at risk for osteoporosis if they have testosterone levels that are so low they result in impotence and absence of nocturnal erections.

The testosterone/bone loss link

A low level of the male sex hormone testosterone, which is common in older men, fosters bone loss. Testosterone is converted to estrogen in the body and, as in women, estrogen is crucial to bone strength in men.

Chronic illness speeds up bone loss

Chronic diseases that affect the kidneys, lungs, stomach, or intestines, or that alter testosterone levels, also place men at a greater than average risk of osteoporosis. Such ailments may require treatments that leach minerals from bone or that interfere with the absorption of bone minerals or their incorporation into bone.

For example, significant bone loss can result from prolonged exposure to cortisone drugs (such as prednisone or others), from anticonvulsant medications, from antacids containing aluminum, as well as some cancer drugs. Aldactone, a diuretic used to treat high blood pressure, can also reduce testosterone levels.

Unofficially... A 16-year study of osteoporosis in men at the Indiana University School of Medicine in Indianapolis found that smoking and drinking outweighed heredity as risk factors for osteoporosis. Most of the men in the Indiana study were so sedentary that it was not possible to make a full assessment of the benefits of physical activity. But the researchers could discern a trend indicating that vigorous activity slowed the rate of bone loss.

But the most prevalent risk factors involve men's smoking and drinking habits, exercise patterns, and diet.

Studies in women have demonstrated that exercising the body's long muscles against gravity—those muscles in the arms, legs, and torso—can actually build new bone, even late in life.

Drink milk!

As for diet, both men and women usually consume inadequate amounts of calcium and vitamin D, which the body needs to absorb and use calcium.

You can easily incorporate high-calcium food choices each day, but you have to plan ahead. Be sure to write these foods on your weekly grocery list, and have them on hand for meal preparation. The food items listed in Table 8.9 and Table 8.10 are inexpensive and easy ways to boost the calcium in your daily diet.

TABLE 8.9: BONE BOOSTING FOODS

Low-fat or non-fat fruit yogurt	Bagel with cheese
Bean and cheese burrito	Calcium-enriched cereal and skim milk
Calcium-enriched juices	Cheeseburger
Cheese pizza	Cheese toast or cheese sandwich using calcium-enriched bread
Cheese sauces over pasta	Chicken Parmesan and noodles
Creamed soups	Dairy sherbet
Fresh vegetables topped with sprinkles of shredded cheese	Frozen yogurt pops
High-calcium cottage cheese with chopped vegetables	High-calcium cottage cheese
Hot chocolate made with 8 ounces milk	Ice milk
Macaroni and cheese	Milkshake

Rice pudding (made with milk)	Romaine salad with shredded cheese on top
Salmon, with bones	Sardines (with bones) and crackers
Sliced cheese and crackers	Sliced toast made with calcium-enriched bread
Spinach quiche	Stuffed shells (romano and mozzarella cheese) with sauce
Taco with cheese	Yogurt

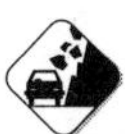

Watch Out!
As we age, the amount of vitamin D made in the skin after exposure to sunlight declines, and the body loses some of its ability to convert vitamin D into the active hormone needed for proper calcium metabolism.

TABLE 8.10: TOP TEN VEGETABLES LOADED WITH CALCIUM

Artichokes	Broccoli	Brussels sprouts
Cabbage	Carrots	Celery
Lima beans	Snap beans	Spinach
Swiss chard		

Consider calcium supplements

If you do not normally drink milk or if you are allergic to it, increase your calcium intake by choosing foods from the list of calcium supplements in Table 8.11.

TABLE 8.11: COMMON CALCIUM SUPPLEMENTS

Alkamints tablets	Biocal calcium tablets	Biocal calcium tablets
Calcium carbonate, liquid	Calcium carbonate tablets	Calcium gluconate tablets
Calcium lactate tablets	Cal-Sup tablets	Caltrate 600 tablets
Caltrate 600+ tablets	Caltrate 600+ D tablets	Digel tablets
Posture tablets	Titralac tablets	Tums tablets
Tums E-X tablets	Tums Ultra tablets	

Treating Osteoporosis without Risk of Impotence

As with women, heredity plays a role in the susceptibility of men to osteoporosis. Men with blood relatives who have developed osteoporosis and had

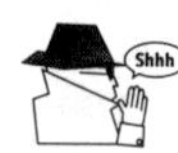

Unofficially... Men need from 1,000 to 1,500 mg of calcium per day for bone strength.

osteoporotic fractures are at greater risk than those with relatives who aged without significant signs of bone loss. While there is nothing a man can do about the three most common risk factors for osteoporosis —age, heredity and being Caucasian—he can certainly modify habits that promote bone loss. That means quitting smoking and limiting alcohol intake to one or two drinks a day, the amount believed to protect the heart. Regular exercise to build fitness and strength, through aerobic workouts and lifting weights or using resistance machines, is also important in preventing the disease.

But to stay strong, bones need the proper raw materials, primarily calcium and vitamin D. In fact, you need to be sure you get:

- 1,000 mg a day of calcium before age 65
- 1,500 mg after age 65
- 400 I.U. a day of vitamin D.

The best, and best-absorbed, sources of these nutrients are low–fat and nonfat dairy products, specifically the daily equivalent of four 8-ounce glasses of skim milk or milk with 1% fat.

Other good sources include sardines and canned salmon (be sure to eat the bones) and some dark-green leafy vegetables, especially collard greens. Those who cannot improve their diets adequately should consider taking a calcium supplement or drinking calcium-fortified orange juice or milk. Supplements of calcium citrate or calcium gluconate are good sources. Calcium carbonate, the ingredient in Tums, is absorbed well enough to help maintain bones.

Medical treatments

Once osteoporosis develops, there are several possible treatments, although none of them have been specifically approved for men. These include calcitonin, through a nasal spray or injections, and alendronate, an oral drug. Men with testosterone deficiency can receive replacement therapy.

As with arthritis, if you are not taking any of the medications to treat your osteoporosis and your doctor feels it's safe, a trial of Viagra might improve erection problems associated with the pain of osteoporosis. If you still have erectile dysfunction, check with your doctor or urologist to see which of the other treatments is best for you.

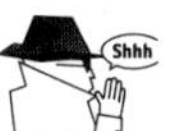

Unofficially... Investors and analysts expect that the market for osteoporosis treatments alone could reach $4 billion a year—with the potential for billions more if the same drugs also prove effective against cancer and Alzheimer's.

New treatments mean fewer side effects

Today the choices for treating arthritis and osteoporosis are many. Revolutionary arthritis drugs that don't carry the dangerous and debilitating side effects of most pain medications will be introduced in 1999, and osteoporosis "cures," such as Fosamax, are being tested on men to see if these will help build bone in the opposite sex.

As stated earlier in this chapter, the most common type of arthritis, osteoarthritis, increases with age and affects millions of Americans. Research shows these newer drugs may also relieve the severe and less common rheumatoid arthritis—as well as reduce the risk of colon cancer and Alzheimer's disease—because they actively reduce inflammation.

Whatever medication you take for arthritis and osteoporosis, keep in mind that you may have side effects. But it's also important to know that such side effects as impotence can now be treated either with Viagra or other options.

Talk with your doctor. Try to use natural methods for keeping your bones, muscles, and joints strong. If you need medication, find the best medication that relieves pain without causing serious side effects.

Just the Facts

- Both arthritis and osteoporosis can make it painful to enjoy sex, yet both can be successfully treated!
- Anti-inflammatory medications can cause impotence as a side effect.
- Men need to have 1,000 to 1,500 mg of calcium in their daily diet through foods or supplements.

Chapter 9

GET THE SCOOP ON...

Erectile dysfunction as a side effect of prescription medications ■ Specific prescriptions that may cause impotence ■ Lowering your dose or changing to a similar medication may stop impotence ■ Antidepressants least likely to affect erectile function

The Nitty-Gritty on Drugs and Medicines

Even though medications are necessary for controlling medical problems, impotence may result as a side effect. It is thought that 25 percent of erectile dysfunction cases are caused by prescription medications. In fact, as many as 200 prescription drugs are known to cause impotence.

If you take medication and also suffer with impotence, your prescription may be the cause. The most common "offending" medications include:

- Diuretics
- Blood pressure medications
- Tranquilizers
- Antidepressants
- Sedatives
- Psychiatric drugs

Surprisingly, there are even many over-the-counter medicines that can cause erectile dysfunction—alcohol, nicotine, and illegal drugs such as cocaine, marijuana, and LSD can also lead to impotence.

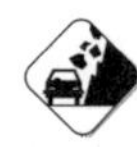

Watch Out!
Never stop taking your medication or change the dosage unless directed by your physician.

The Medicine/Impotence Link

If you develop erectile dysfunction while taking a medication, that medication may be the culprit. In many cases, it is common for this medication/impotence link to go undetected because, quite honestly, most men do not like to talk about sexual function with their doctor or pharmacist. And the chances that your doctor would ask you about erectile problems during a routine medical check-up are slim to none. Even if your doctor did inquire about erection problems, most men would find the topic too embarrassing and end the discussion.

A recent connection

Research has only recently started to focus on how drugs—even life-saving medications—can affect a patient's quality of life, including his sexual life. Therefore, even many doctors are not fully aware of the medication/impotence link.

In numerous cases, once a patient discovers that a medication can affect his sexual function, it is common for him to stop the medication on his own. This can lead to other, very serious problems. For example, if you are taking blood pressure medication, including diuretics, for a problem like hypertension, stopping this medication to increase your erectile function could cause you greater problems down the road. It could even put you at risk of heart attack or stroke. That is why open communication with your doctor about this common problem is crucial. Keep in mind that the solutions are varied and often as simple as a change in medications.

How medications affect sexual function

Years ago, men with severe hypertension almost always had to choose between controlling their blood pressure or having erections and sexual activity. For millions of men, this was an easy choice. They simply ignored the hypertension and chose to enjoy sex. The choice, however, carried a high price, because after many years of doing this, the result was early heart disease or stroke.

Fortunately, having to make this difficult choice is no longer necessary because there are now many medications that control hypertension without the side effect of erectile dysfunction. Complementary choices such as a diet high in fruits and vegetables and low in saturated fat, daily exercise, and stress reduction can also help.

Some medications can affect sexual function and erection by making us sleepy or changing our personality. Some can even cause us to lose interest in sex. Tranquilizers and sedatives may alter your personality, even though the medication itself should not cause problems.

Since everyone is different, even medications that do not usually cause erectile dysfunction in most patients might be affecting you in your own situation. If these are not considered, you may go years without realizing that a simple change in medication can change your entire sexual life.

Bright Idea
Brown bag it. To make sure your doctor knows all your medications, vitamins, and supplements, pack them in a paper bag and take them with you when you next visit your doctor. This will help him make sure that you will not have a drug/drug interaction, as well as determine that you are not taking a medication that may be causing impotence.

Get it out on the table

In most cases, you've got to talk about your erectile problems with your doctor. You need to discuss the medications you are taking, and even bring these to your doctor's office so he can evaluate the side effects of various chemicals.

It may take a bit of trial and error—and a lot of patience—to find the correct combination of medications to treat your other medical problems while also curing your impotence. Since medications are

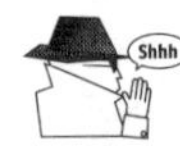

Unofficially... It is estimated that 10 to 30 percent of men who take medications for blood pressure may suffer sexual problems, mainly erectile dysfunction.

used to treat real health problems, keep in mind that many problems, as discussed in Part II of this book, contribute to erectile dysfunction and can make it even more difficult to identify the side effect of a particular dose of medication.

High Blood Pressure Medications... Low Sex Function

Certain groups of blood pressure medications commonly cause impotence. In some men, these medications can be taken with great success and no side effects are experienced. Yet in others, while the hypertension is controlled, these medications also cause impotence.

Some of the most common examples of these drugs are listed in Table 9.1. You may find that a drug given by tablet might cause erection problems, yet the same drug given by skin patch might be problem-free.

TABLE 9.1: COMMONLY USED HYPERTENSION DRUGS THAT MAY CAUSE IMPOTENCE

Accupril*	Aldactazide	Aldactone	Aldomet
Aldoril	Altace*	Apresazide	Apresoline*
Blocadren	Cartrol	Catapres	Capoten*
Corgard	Dibenzaline	Diupres	Diuril
Dyazide	Esidrix	Eutonyl	Hydrodiuril
Hydropres	Hygroton	Inderal	Inderide
Ismelin	Levatol	Lotensin*	Lopressor
Lozol	Maxzide	Metatensin	Midamor
Minipress*	Moduretic	Monopril*	Normodyne
Oretic	Regitine	Regroton	Salutensin
Sectral	Ser-Ap-Es	Serpasil	Tenex
Tenormin	Toprol	Thiazides	Vasotec*
Visken	Wytensin	Zaroxolyn	Zebeta
Ziac	Zestril*		

*Least likely to cause impotence

Heart Disease and Sexual Activity

Heart disease can by itself make sexual activity more difficult. In fact, the combination of heart disease and cigarette smoking has been found by some researchers to be a strong cause of erectile dysfunction.

Hypertension medications add to the problems of heart disease because they can increase the side effects you may experience. (Many medications used for hypertension are also used to help in heart problems.)

Many medications used for heart disease can by themselves cause erection problems. Digoxin is an older medication and an established treatment that improves the pumping function of the heart and controls irregular or fast heart rate. However, in some men, it can result in reduced sexual activity and erectile dysfunction.

Other medications, such as Norpace beta-blockers, which are used to control irregular heart rate and other rhythm problems, can cause erectile dysfunction.

Although there are a number of these medications available, in an individual patient one specific medication may be necessary to control the heart rhythm problem. Being aware that erection problems can occur with these drugs will help you and your doctor choose the one that heals with the least possible side effects.

Less Anxiety May Mean Less Sex

Drugs used to treat anxiety can actually improve sexual function and erection if they help reduce the anxiety that is creating this problem. This is especially true when they are used in low doses. Yet in higher doses, these same drugs may cause further depression, thus creating more sexual problems. Some newer drugs such as buspirone have rarely been associated with erectile dysfunction.

Which came first?

Since depression can itself cause decreased sexual activity and erectile dysfunction, effective treatment with medications can improve sexual activity, commonly with a corresponding improvement in erectile function. However, many of the older antidepressants can cause erectile dysfunction, especially when used in higher doses.

Bright Idea
Ask your doctor to try some of the newer cholesterol-lowering medications. Some of the older medications used to lower abnormal cholesterol levels can cause erectile dysfunction, yet newer drugs may not affect you sexually.

Newer drugs may bring relief

The newer antidepressant drugs, called SSRIs (selective serotonin reuptake inhibitors), have improved the treatment of depression and lowered many of the side effects. Just as with the other antidepressant drugs, when your depression is improved, there also may be improvement in erection problems. Some of the SSRIs, however, can also cause sexual dysfunction including erectile dysfunction. Changing to another one of this group of drugs, the problem may be helped. Some men find that stopping these medications for short periods, such as on weekends, helps diminish the unwanted effects on sexual function. Always consult your doctor before adjusting your dosage in this manner. Another possibility is adding a medication, such as yohimbine, if your doctor approves, to offset the negative effect on erections, while allowing the antidepressant to be continued. Since each person is different, talk with your doctor to see which plan is most likely to help you without side effects.

Some other antidepressants have been associated with fewer side effects on sexual function and may improve sexual performance, especially if there already was an impotence problem. These include Wellbutrin, Effexor, Serzone, and Luvox.

TABLE 9.2: COMMONLY USED ANTI-ANXIETY MEDICATIONS THAT MAY CAUSE IMPOTENCE

Buspar	Equanil	Equagesic	Lentrex
Librium	Miltown	Serax	Tranxene
Triavil	Tybatran	Ritalin	Valium
Valrelease	Xanax		

TABLE 9.3: COMMONLY USED ANTIDEPRESSANTS THAT MAY CAUSE IMPOTENCE

Anafranil	Aventyl	Celexa	Efrafon
Elavil	Endet	Ludiomil	Marplan
Nardil	Norpramin	Pamelor	Parnate
Paxil	Pertofrane	Prozac	Sinequan
Surmontil	Tofranil	Vivactil	Zoloft

TABLE 9.4: COMMONLY USED TRANQUILIZERS THAT MAY CAUSE IMPOTENCE

Haldol	Innovar	Mellaril	Navane
Prolixin	Serentil	Sparine	Stelazine
Taractan	Thorazine		

Other Medications That Cause Impotence

There are still many other medications that may affect your erectile function; more than 200 known drugs cause impotence. The following drugs are reported to cause erectile dysfunction:

- Lithium used for bipolar disorder, depression
- Eskalith
- Lithobid
- Lithonate
- Lithotab

TABLE 9.5: OTHER COMMONLY USED DRUGS THAT MAY CAUSE IMPOTENCE

Drugs for Parkinson's Disease:			
Akineton	Artane	Cogentin	Kemadrin
Laradopa	Sinemet	Pagitane	
Antihistamines:			
Ambenyl	Antivert	Atarax	Benadryl
Benylin	Bonine	Bromanyl	Dituss
Dramamine	Mepergan	Nico-vent	Phenergan
Synalgos	Vistaril		
Muscle Relaxants:			
Flexeril	Norflex	Norgesin	
Miscellaneous:			
Accutane	Amicar	Atromid-S	Axid
Cogentia	Copazine	Dilantin	Donnatol
Estrace	Estrogens	Eulitin	Fastin
Flagyl	Furoxone	Glucocortico	Lanoxin
Lopid	Lupron	Mutulane	Mysoline
Nizoral	Norpace	Pepcid	Phenobarbital
Pro-Banthine	Proscar	Reglan	Sansert
Tagamet	Tegretol	Timoptic eye drops	Zantac
Zoladex	Immunosuppressive agents		

TABLE 9.6: COMMONLY ABUSED DRUGS THAT MAY CAUSE IMPOTENCE

Alcohol	Amyl nitrate ("poppers")	Amphetamines	Barbiturates
Cocaine	Heroin	Marijuana	Methadone
Morphine	Nicotine in cigarettes	Opiates	PCP ("angel dust")

Taking Charge of Your Health

Even though your doctor may say that a specific drug should not cause erectile dysfunction, if you notice this as a side effect, bring it to your doctor's attention. We are all different, and everyone reacts differently to medication. See if your doctor will change the dosage or try a different medication until you find one that works to treat your problem, as well as leave you without impotence.

Just the Facts

- The realization that medications could affect erectile function is a relatively new discovery.
- Wellbutrin, Effexor, Serzone, and Luvox are newer antidepressants that are least likely to affect erectile function.
- Sometimes simply changing the dosage of your medication will correct the impotence.

PART III

The Truth About Psychological Causes

Chapter 10

GET THE SCOOP ON...
Impotence and emotional health ▪ Stress, the brain, and erectile function ▪ How to tell if you may be a workaholic ▪ Performance anxiety and impotence

The Psychological Dilemma

If you are impotent, chances are great that there are also psychological implications. This does not mean that this problem is permanent or even threatening to your overall emotional health. What this does mean is that any man who does not feel he can function as a male—even if the problem is caused by the physical problems discussed in this book—will feel frayed, fragile, and psychologically weak. The good news is that once your impotence is corrected or reversed, the psychological barrier usually goes away.

Consider this: During sex, a woman can pretend to be aroused, even if she is not. If she is worried, distracted, or even stressed out, she can still fake arousal or even an orgasm. Chances are great that few men can honestly tell if a woman is fully aroused or just pretending.

Yet how can a man fake an erection? He can't. When he fails to perform during sex because of impotence, it is obvious and usually humiliating.

Bright Idea
You can discern if your impotence is psychological or physical by using the postage-stamp test. Glue a strip of postage stamps around the shaft of your penis before you go to bed. If the strip is intact in the morning, you have not had any erections during sleep, meaning something is wrong with the mechanics of the system.

Even when a man is sexually "turned on" and wants to be fully involved in making love, the outward "sign" of erectile dysfunction sends another message to his partner.

Not only is erectile dysfunction embarrassing, but frequently the failure to have a full erection is frightening and brings on a host of psychological problems, such as anxiety, fear, and, in some cases, even depression. You may feel that you are no longer worthy as a husband or lover. Or, you may feel that you are now "over the hill," as so many men correlate increasing years with decreasing sexual function.

None of this is true! Impotence is very common, and while it does cause anxiety and feelings of emotional vulnerability, it is also easy to correct in most cases.

The Stress/Impotence Connection

You may not want to hear this, but stress is here to stay, and stress may be the cause of your impotence. Whether your stress comes from a demanding career, aggressive drivers during rush hour, more month than money, or family situations that are out of control—stress can literally sneak up on you and drain you of all your energy. Most of the time you don't even realize you are stressed out until you are suffering from some stress-related problem.

It's probably no news to you that most men today work 24 hours a day, seven days a week—even when they are not supposed to be "at work." A recent poll by the Gallup Organization revealed that for more than half of those age 35 to 54—stress is a familiar part of their daily lives. Job and financial problems were the leading stressors. For many men in white-collar jobs, even downtime is spent negotiating deals with clients on cellular phones or answering faxes and e-mail at home.

A simple definition

To help you understand how stress affects your performance in the bedroom, let's first analyze what constitutes stress. Simply stated, stress describes the many demands and pressures that all people experience to some degree each day. These demands may be physical, mental, emotional, or even chemical in nature. The word we call "stress" includes both the stressful situation known as the "stressor," and the symptoms you experience under stress, called the "stress response."

Keep in mind that just about anything you encounter can cause stress. Usually it is not life's emergencies or disasters that trigger the majority of stress reactions, but more often it is the persistent interruptions, struggles, and irritating hassles you face every day. Whether you are confronted with financial or health problems, waiting in long lines of traffic each evening, or raising rebellious teens, all of these can add up to overwhelming stress. Likewise, the stress can also result in a glitch or malfunction in the brain/penis connection and subsequently cause erectile dysfunction.

So, how often do you feel stressed? Some men with impotence tell of also feeling too much stress around the same time. A recent survey found that 16 percent of those questioned felt stressed "all the time" and could not seem to relax, while 52 percent of those questioned felt stressed "most of the time."

Every week, an estimated 95 million Americans suffer a stress-related problem and take medication for their aches and pains. There are estimates that as much as 80 percent of all illness is stress-related, and 85 percent of all industrial accidents are linked to worker behavior that includes adaptation to

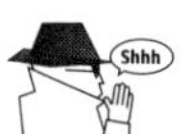

Unofficially...
Using data from the Massachusetts Male Aging Study, researchers found that impotence is nearly twice as likely in men with depressive symptoms compared with those without such symptoms.

stress. In new data from a study done by the Massachusetts Institute of Technology Analysis Group, researchers estimate that depression, which can be triggered by ongoing stress, costs American business $43.7 billion a year, an expense equal to that of heart disease.

> "I feel stressed every minute of every day."
> —Ben, air traffic controller, 46

Stress can cause a wide variety of physical changes and emotional responses—such as erectile dysfunction. Stress symptoms vary greatly from one person to the next, and learning to identify the ways in which your body and mind react to stress is an important step in treating and managing this problem.

The different stages of stress

As many researchers have explained, with stress, perception is absolutely paramount. Unless you think that something is going to be a threat, it is not going to trigger the stress response that comes when you realize that there is a potential threat.

To understand how perception can increase your stress response, consider the differences between good friends. For example, your best friend may look forward to going to the local fair on his day off and jumping off a platform with a bungee cord attached to his body. For him, this is an amazingly exhilarating experience and gives him a rush of adrenaline and emotional excitement. Conversely, the thought of bungee jumping may cause you more anxiety than an IRS audit.

It's important to understand that while the environmental trigger is identical, different people perceive situations in totally different ways. Different individuals also have different susceptibilities to stress. It is true that we all need a certain amount of emotional excitement in our lives to counter the effects of boredom and tedium. Driving your car to work during rush hour may be all the emotional excitement you need. Yet your friend may have a very high threshold for emotional excitement and achieves it by skydiving or by participating in other high-risk sports. Your threshold for responding to stress is dictated largely in your genetic blueprint.

No matter what causes your stress, when you are exposed to a stressful situation perceived as threatening, your body prepares for confrontation. The response is physical and is controlled by your hormones and nervous system and is known as the "fight or flight response." You are prepared to fight or flee your stressor—yes, even the dog barking at midnight is a stressor! Even though we no longer need to fight wild animals, those wild animals exist metaphorically as long lines of traffic, fights with friends or family members, or just hearing a telephone ring constantly day after day. When confronted with a stressful situation, such as an unexpected bill or a reprimand by your boss, your body produces adrenaline. The release of adrenaline is like sending a thousand telegrams to different parts of your body all at once. These telegrams prepare your body to deal with the stress, whether positive or negative.

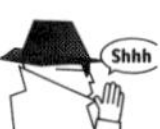

Unofficially... Hans Selye, an endocrinologist and biologist, was one of the first scientists to explain stress and its effects on our bodies, saying that stress is "the non-specific response of the body to any demand." In his book *Stress Without Distress*, Selye describes the physiological response to stressors in three stages known as the General Adaptation Syndrome (GAS).

Loss of control increases stress response

You probably think you can deal with any amount of stress. After all, you are a man, and men are supposed to be strong. Right? Not really. Feeling that you are no longer in control can cause fear and anxiety—in both men and women. Think about how you might feel at the zoo. You may be watching a caged lion from behind a fence—a protective barrier. However, the moment that barrier is removed, that animal becomes a threat. Being in control is similar to that protective barrier. It is when the sense of control is lost and you feel helpless that anxiety and subsequent health problems will occur.

Bright Idea
If you are undergoing a stressful period, try to fill your life with positive stress (eustress) to counteract the negative effect of stress (distress) by having a party, going on vacation, or even simply taking yourself out for a good meal. Relaxation would be even better.

Consider the first time you experienced erectile dysfunction. You probably felt like your world had caved in—your body had failed you. You went from fully functioning as a man should sexually to not functioning at all. This type of loss of control can make your heart race and blood pressure rise. And the fear that this condition will continue can cause you even more anxiety. This stress could further compound your impotence problem.

As discussed above, no matter what causes the stress, it will show itself through a wide variety of physical changes and emotional responses. These symptoms vary greatly from one person to the next. Perhaps the most universal sign of stress is a feeling of being pressured or overwhelmed.

Stress symptoms vary greatly from one person to the next, but in addition to feeling pressured or overwhelmed, look at Table 10.1 and see which symptoms apply to your situation.

TABLE 10.1: COMMON STRESS SYMPTOMS

Anger	Anxiety	Apathy
Back pain	Chest pains	Tightness in chest
Colitis	Depression	Heart palpitations
Hives	IBS (irritable bowel syndrome)	Impotence
Inability to relax at night	Inability to concentrate	Jaw pain
Migraine headaches	Loss of sexual desire	
Neck pain	No energy	Rapid pulse
Rashes	Short temper	Short-term memory loss
Tension headaches	Weight loss	Weight gain

If you are experiencing a few of these symptoms, chances are that your level of stress is excessive. If left untreated, stress can lead to permanent feelings of helplessness, ineffectiveness, and possibly depression. An acute or prolonged tense state may cause increased heart rate and blood pressure, dry mouth, enlarged pupils, sweaty palms, and fast, shallow "chest" breathing.

How stress causes impotence

The ongoing stress and anxiety from marital, financial, or other external problems can psychologically affect your sexual performance. Stress contributes to increased blood pressure and cholesterol, thereby contributing to a greater risk of impotence. For example, you may have had no problem performing sexually until you lost your job or received a pay cut. In this regard, it is possible for your high level of worry, anxiety, and stress to interfere with nerve impulses in your brain when you attempt sexual intercourse. This happens because stress causes an adrenaline release that sets up a whole cascade of reactions including increased heart rate and blood pressure. The brain thus receives all sorts of mixed or negative signals from the body, causing the brain/penis connection to short-circuit.

To experience erectile dysfunction for the first time can cause a great deal of anxiety, but repeated failure to "function as a man" can lead to a cycle of anxiety that only perpetuates the problem, making sexual activity impossible. It works something like this:

1) Stress causes you to experience erectile dysfunction.

2) The fear that you will again fail causes performance anxiety,

3) which creates more stress,

4) which perpetuates the erectile dysfunction,

5) which in turn creates even more stress.

And so it goes. Performance anxiety can thus perpetuate impotence, causing it to occur again—and again and again, creating a never-ending cycle of sexual frustration.

Overachiever or Underachiever?

As you begin to think about the stress you face, and what steps you must take to lessen this risk factor for impotence, it's important to evaluate your life and consider new ways to balance it. Do you know anyone who said on his deathbed that he wished he had spent more time at the office? Fortunately, you don't have to wait until then to realize you may need to make some changes if you want to enjoy some of life's pleasures, like a sexual relationship with someone you love.

It's easy to recognize the compulsive and addictive behavior of alcoholics, drug addicts, and gamblers. You may even acknowledge that other "normal" behaviors such as watching sports on TV, obsessive shopping, or cleanliness, or the uncontrollable need to exercise, while not addictive, can all create problems requiring help when they are practiced in excess.

What motivates workaholics?

However, what about the long hours you work? We know that you would probably argue that you do so because you have financial or other obligations. "A problem from working too much? Not me!" you might say. You may even deny that working too many hours is compulsive or addictive. Yet you may be surprised to know that being a workaholic is addictive, compulsive, and can interfere with the rest of your life, including your ability to perform sexually.

Perhaps you come from a family where being successful is valued and promoted. You may have lived with the fear of not being good enough or of disappointing someone close to you. In this regard, these inner feelings will literally drive you to keep working in order to hide your real feelings of inadequacy.

"There's no way I'm a workaholic. I'm successful, highly motivated, and responsible." This may all be true. Outwardly, these appear as positive values—the American Work Ethic. Yet inwardly, if carried to the extreme, workaholics may actually be masking underlying fears and insecurities.

Through hard work, the workaholic has found a method of altering feelings that are painful and confusing. These may be the fear of failing, of being victimized, or of losing control, among many.

The mood-altering experience of workaholism becomes so intense and captivating that it takes on a life of its own. It becomes difficult or impossible to control, and it dramatically affects others.

"Through my years of counseling, I've noted that some overachievers in the boardroom are underachievers in the bedroom."
—Samantha, sex therapist, 47

No time for love

Sometimes when workaholics experience sexual dysfunction, it stems from something more than an inability to achieve an erection. You may have serious problems in keeping and maintaining an intimate relationship with your spouse or lover simply because you have not put time into it.

Your spouse may be exhibiting codependent behavior similar to the alcoholic's spouse, giving a host of excuses or rationalizations as to why you do not attend dinner parties, movies, or other outings with friends and family. She may have convinced herself that you do not perform sexually because you are just "too tired" from the demands at your workplace.

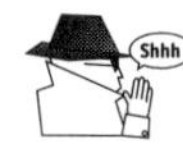

Unofficially... Research has identified four key elements that contribute to a workaholic's degree of happiness:

1. The acceptance of their work habits by their families.
2. The amount of autonomy and variety in their work.
3. The good match between their personal skills and those required by their work.
4. Their good state of health.

Workaholic or love to work?

Simply having some of the symptoms or reflecting some of the characteristics mentioned above does not necessarily mean you are a bona fide workaholic. You could be one of the many men who absolutely loves what you do. You may work hard, put in many hours at the workplace, but you also balance this heavy workload with an enthusiasm for life—filled with friends and family and activities separate from work. The healthy worker uses his career or work to enhance his life and relationships. The workaholic uses work to survive. Sometimes it takes someone other than yourself to see the difference, but check out the list below to see if any of these warning signs apply to you:

- You thrive on overtime.
- You look forward to those 12 to 15 hours a day at the office.
- You always have a briefcase full of papers to review.
- You need to stay up after everyone has gone to bed to finish one more project.
- You haven't had a vacation in years.
- The last time you took a vacation, you could not wait to get home and get back to work.
- You never take the time to enjoy family outings.
- You dread Sundays and cannot wait for Monday morning to arrive.

- You have a hard time relaxing.
- At home, your thoughts are on what needs to be done at the office.
- At the office, you rarely think about your needs at home.
- You frequently feel pressure or anger about money.
- Your spouse and kids don't really know you anymore.
- You do not know your family very well.
- You have not been sexually intimate with your spouse in months.
- Your kids are having problems in school.
- You are not feeling appreciated or understood.
- You may be eating and/or drinking too much.
- You may be thinking about or wishing for an affair.
- You promise to slow down, but never do.
- When you do take time to be sexually intimate, you find that you are impotent.

> "According to the Institute of Organizational Health at the Washington Business Group on Health, the inflexible addiction to work is what is unhealthy."

It's in the personality

Your specific personality type can have a profound impact upon susceptibility to becoming a workaholic. You have probably heard of the so-called Type A personality. These people are literally slaves to the clock. They are always in a hurry and seldom take time out to enjoy life. They are time-oriented and frequently speak with a very rapid rate of speech, finishing the sentences of those they are speaking to as they grow impatient. This is in marked contrast to the Type B personality, who is quite simply a non-Type A. The Type B individual gets the work done, but he also takes time out to smell the roses.

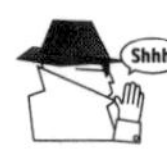

Unofficially... A study reported in The Lancet suggests that long commutes and extended work hours may over-activate the sympathetic nervous system, which kicks in the fight or flight response. If you are fighting wild animals, this response is normal. However, the increase in the production of stress hormones will only serve to tear down your immune function.

It was initially concluded that it was the Type A individual who was most likely to succumb to a heart attack. That conclusion is still to be found in many basic psychology textbooks. Yet that is only partly true. Researchers now believe that it is not so much the time orientation that is responsible for the associated heart problems, but rather the negative emotions associated with stress. For example, anger and hostility account for the correlation between the Type A personality and heart disease. In other words, it is probably okay to be a workaholic, but just don't be an angry, hostile workaholic!

The Type C or cancer-prone personality has been associated with certain forms of cancer. This individual is strikingly similar to the so-called rheumatoid arthritic personality, a term coined by Dr. George Solomon in the mid-1960s. Both individuals are extremely passive and are willing to endure a great deal of personal discomfort to please other people. It is the person who will frequently say "yes" when he really wants to say "no." There may be many reasons why this individual is more vulnerable to infections and certain forms of cancer, but one may be related to the issue of control. In a sense, people who allow their actions to be dictated by others are not in control of their lives. In extreme cases, they form co-dependent relationships with others that can be extremely unhealthy for both members of the relationship.

A final type of personality is the so-called Type T, or thrill-seeking, personality. Medical science is not aware of any classic diseases associated with taking risks, although these individuals do have a decreased life expectancy because of the risks that they do take. It is noteworthy, however, that most drug addicts have Type T or thrill-seeking personalities. This fits with the hypothesis of many mental health workers that many addicts are addicted not only to the chemical formulations that they abuse, but also to the risk associated with living on the edge. They become addicted to the thrill associated with stealing to support their habit or perhaps even the risk associated with the changes in their health.

Now before you quit your job and try to change your workaholic, Type A personality, keep reading. There is no such thing as a "pure" type A, B, C, or T personality. While it is true that our genetic code and early experiences can have a profound impact on our ultimate personality, the environment in which we find ourselves is equally important. There is a certain amount of overlap among the various model personalities. For example, you may be a classic Type A personality at work, a Type B when at home with your family, and then a Type C when you check into the hospital. In other words, you might be a composite of all these personalities. It does turn out, though, that most of the time you will exhibit the characteristics of one or just a couple of these personality constructs.

While this is a useful way to categorize people, it might be more accurate to think of "personalities" as coping styles that enable people to deal with problems in their immediate environment. These are just a few of the many factors that can affect how your body responds to life's stressors.

Finding balance

When working too long and too hard each day increases the stress in your life, you place yourself at great risk for impotence. Keep in mind that many overachievers in the workplace are underachievers in the bedroom.

> "Did you know that STRESSED spelled backwards is DESSERTS?"
> —Mary Ann, certified nutritionist, 34

Talk with your doctor about your work habits if you feel you have many of the warning signs of a workaholic, and using the Relaxation Response in Chapter 13 and other tips for stress reduction, to get your life back in balance.

When Stressed Becomes Depressed

Long-term stress can often cause situational or chronic symptoms of depression. Perhaps you do not feel depressed and outwardly you may seem quite happy. But when you live with sleepless nights and worries about your body seemingly failing you, as many with impotence do, depression should be considered. The symptoms of depression, which are listed in Table 10.2, are many and varied:

TABLE 10.2: COMMON SIGNS AND SYMPTOMS OF DEPRESSION

Disturbances in sleep patterns	Fatigue
Loss of interest in usual activities	Impaired thinking
Thoughts of dying or suicide	Mood swings
Depressed thoughts or irritable moods	Difficulty concentrating
Loss of interest in activities such as hobbies	Staying at home all the time
Avoidance of special friends	Excessive sleep
Lack of sleep	Reduced or increased appetite
Weight loss or gain (more than five percent of body weight)	

From mild sadness to major episodes

Depression comes in several forms, a chronic, low-grade depression called *dysthymia* to a major depressive episode. People experiencing that latter emotion may express such symptoms as uncontrollable tearfulness, feelings of helplessness and/or hopelessness, loss of self-worth, and suicidal thoughts. If you have these feelings, contact a professional to get help.

In the book *From Sad to Glad* author Nathan S. Kline said that depression might be defined as the magnified and inappropriate expression of some otherwise quite common emotional responses. That, of course, is true of many other disorders. By way of analogy, one expects to find heart palpitations in a person who has just run up a steep hill. Something is decidedly amiss, however, if such palpitation occurs during a sedate walk.

So, too, with depression. All of us experience moments of sadness, loneliness, pessimism, and uncertainty as a natural reaction to particular circumstances. Yet in the depressed person these feelings become all-pervasive; they can be triggered by the smallest incident or occur without evident connection to any outside cause. At times there may be a sudden burst of tears that the person cannot explain, while others may experience a more or less constant weepiness.

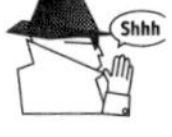

Unofficially... Dysthymia is defined as being in a depressed mood more days than not for at least two years.

How you may feel

Depression generally occurs when negative thoughts compound upon themselves and get so rooted into the subconscious that you cannot break out of the cycle of negativism and self-pity. If left untreated, depression can last for months or even years, leading to feelings of helplessness and, at worst, suicide. It is not a sign of personal weakness or moral corruption. You can no more pull yourself together and get over depression than you can will away diabetes or cancer.

The problem with depression is that not only is it debilitating, it can ruin your life.

Although most researchers find that twice as many women succumb to depression as men, it still happens to men and can affect their performance at home, in the boardroom, and in the bedroom.

Many times depression can stem from a biochemical imbalance or can be the symptom of an underlying ailment. And quite often, professional medical help, and the use of medication and therapy, is needed to maintain, control, and cure depression. There are many excellent prescription drugs and many medical protocols that can assist you if this is the case.

Help is available

If you feel depression is a concern, see a qualified mental health specialist. Studies show that up to 85 percent of patients will find relief through treatment with antidepressant medications, psychotherapy, or electroshock therapy. Again, if you are having suicidal thoughts, take these seriously and seek professional help.

Keep in mind that alcohol and drugs cannot combat depression. While the medication your doctor prescribes is specially formulated to balance your body's chemicals, alcohol and other drugs may worsen your situation. Make sure that you only use medication prescribed by your physician.

As you will read in Chapter 14, exercise is a great cure for easing mild depression. Determine what you can do physically, and start a program. Physical activities can increase mental alertness and increase the endorphins (the body's natural opiates), which will give you a calming, contented feeling.

Be sure to stick to a routine each day. Staying in bed all day, unless advised by your doctor, cannot help you alleviate the depressive feelings. Also, consider reaching out to others to get out of your own problems.

When Hopelessness Hits

Sometimes being impotent can affect your pride. It can lead to decreased intimacy with your spouse or person you love. For many men, their self-esteem is wrapped up in the ability to perform like a man in every way—including sexually. Men who think in this way, and are unable to perform sexually, are likely to see themselves as failures.

When we feel badly about ourselves or focus on what we can't do, our outlook on life takes on a negative perspective. When this happens, small problems appear to be insurmountable. Although you most likely have had some failures before in life, being impotent may be the first one to make you feel like less of a man. This may be the first major ego-threatening problem you have ever had to face.

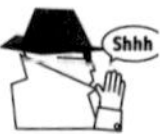

Unofficially... As many as 12 to 14 million Americans are affected with depression each year, and this figure extends to as many as 13 to 20 percent of the total population in the United States having depression at any given time.

In addition, other problems associated with impotence can make you feel as if you've lost control of your body. For example, diabetes can cause erectile dysfunction. The medications you may take for high blood pressure can also cause impotence, as can medications taken for anxiety or depression. Yet, if these ailments are not controlled by medications, you will be suffering something far greater than impotence. Uncontrolled diabetes can cause heart disease, blindness, and the destruction of organs. Unmanaged hypertension can lead to heart attack or stroke.

In the midst of hopelessness and feelings of despair, many men turn to drugs and alcohol. While these may briefly numb the pain of depression or anxiety, the effects are often short-lived. You may also be left with the complicated side effects of addiction, depression, and a higher incidence of impotence.

Bright Idea
Be sure to find some humor, joy, and pleasure at least once a day. Try the newspaper cartoons, or even the situation comedies on TV. You should try to have at least one good laugh a day to combat sadness.

When sadness or depression sets in, you may find relief with a few beers at night. However, over a period of time, you will need more alcohol to numb your painful emotional state.

Alcohol is a substance that has to be taken in ever-increasing dosages to adequately dull emotional despair. In addition, it is a depressant that leaves a "down" mood once the effects wear off. Long-term use of alcohol also carries with it the danger of cognitive deficits such as memory difficulties, visual and spatial problems, and decreased motor function. Anxiety or depression is one thing, but damage to the brain is another. It is not a smart trade-off.

In essence, drugs and alcohol are dangerous methods of controlling your "down" moods. Some drugs, such as those your physician prescribes, may be of value, but you should make sure they are safe and without unwanted side effects.

If you think that you might be abusing drugs or alcohol, shed that pride and seek professional help. Likewise, if your family has been asking you to see someone for the problem, do them and yourself a favor—accept the help. If you believe that you are addicted, consider admitting yourself to a detox program.

Coping With the Feelings of Impotence

You may find it frightening to be impotent and even more frightening to think that the condition may continue. You may feel that being impotent and not being able to fully enjoy sex is like having no life at all. Your problem is very real, and it can have a devastating affect on your outlook on life and your daily activities.

Fortunately, it is possible to learn effective strategies for coping with your feelings about impotence. In doing so, you can alleviate stress and unnecessary anxiety.

Coping with anxiety and fear

Many men who are impotent experience feelings of anxiety and fear. These fears are very real. When patients are asked about these fears, they usually respond with questions such as:

- Will my chances of being impotent increase with age?
- How can I handle the anxiety of worrying about being impotent?
- How can I talk openly with my spouse?
- How can I ever enjoy sex again?

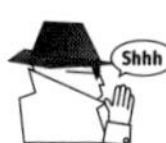

Unofficially... The U.S. market for antidepressants is expected to reach $6 billion in the year 1998.

Obsessing over your fears will make it difficult to find a solution for erectile dysfunction. Remember how the brain has to send a signal to the penis in order for an erection to occur? The more stressed and worried you are about your ability to perform sexually, the greater the chances are that this "connection" will not occur.

It is far better to recognize your fears, talk openly about them with your doctor or spouse, then learn to relax and let go of unnecessary "performance anxieties."

To cope with anxiety and fear:

- Write down the situations that make you anxious and fearful—a certain program or newscast on television, a friend who is negative, conflict with a family member who does not accept your condition, even stories you read in the morning paper. Try to avoid these situations when possible.
- Do not expect your spouse to be your therapist. Find a licensed mental health counselor, and make an appointment to "talk it out" with an impartial trained professional who understands sexual problems.

- Keep an open mind about complementary medical interventions that can help you relax, such as relaxation response, music or laughter therapy, or herbs for relaxation (see Chapter 14).
- Ask your physician to explain the nature of impotence so you understand what you can control and what you cannot. There are many medical treatments available that will help you to move beyond this condition. While you try these treatments, stick with your doctor until you find one that works best in your situation.

> "Worrying about what happened the last time you tried to have sex will only make you more anxious and fearful and will increase the chance that this may occur again." —Charles, urologist, 42

Coping with suspicion

Living with impotence can make you more sensitive to what others say and do. You may feel as if coworkers or friends know you are impotent and take things they may say out of context. Or, you may feel as if your spouse is resentful because of the effect of your impotence on the marriage relationship. Constant, unrelenting fears day after day can result in distorted thoughts. This does not mean that you are crazy! Instead, it means that the stress has affected the way you interpret what people do and say. If you find yourself being overly suspicious, sit back, and consider the possibility that you might be overreacting.

Coping with anger

If you have lived with impotence for months or even years, you may be feeling very angry. Anger is a natural reaction to impotence, but how men express that anger can vary. Some use the anger in a positive manner, some ignore the anger, and some let angry feelings consume their whole beings.

In order to cope with the anger and irritability that often accompanies a failure to perform sexually, it will help to understand the different types of anger. Once you do this, you can replace the energy you spent being angry with positive actions to make life enjoyable for you and those around you. The different types of anger are:

- *Upfront anger.* This is expressed directly toward the person or situation at which you are angry. Used moderately, this is the most acceptable way of expressing anger. It's OK to tell your partner or doctor such things as, "Yes, I hate it that I'm impotent," or "I feel so frustrated and angry when I want to express myself sexually yet am unable to" — so long as you do not follow through with violent outbursts.

- *Displaced anger.* With this type of anger, your strong feelings toward the problem (in this case, impotence), are directed toward a different person or event. For example, rather than telling your wife how angry you are about your impotence, you might instead berate her by saying that her looks or weight are causing your sexual problems. Instead of expressing anger toward the initial problem, you yell at your wife, expressing *displaced anger.* Displaced anger won't solve your problem: it will only cause additional grief as you lose control and lash out at innocent victims.

- *Inward anger.* Instead of speaking openly about your angry thoughts, you let them boil up inside, resulting in physical ailments such as nausea, tension headaches, muscle aches, or even depression. Obviously, this isn't a healthy response.

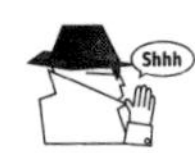

Unofficially... An interesting research study demonstrates how powerful mental interpretation can be. A group of 75-year-old men and women were placed in a retreat for one week and were told to act "55 again." To help complete the illusion, the entire retreat was equipped with items dating back 20 years—old telephones, old magazines, etc. After one week, the seniors showed improved hearing, eyesight, dexterity, and appetites. Their mental ability improved, and believe it or not, they actually measured taller in height!

Coping with worry

Your doctor confirms your greatest fear—yes, you are impotent. All of a sudden you are faced with the reality of growing older, which creates anxiety and fears. Some men worry about the changes that can occur with aging, such as changes in looks, serious illnesses, loss of abilities, loneliness, and death. Many men confuse some of the normal changes in their bodies with changes caused by terminal diseases and obsess on these changes to the point of becoming completely immobilized. Worries about eating the right foods to prevent diseases or about normal changes in senses, such as hearing or sight, begin to add to these other health anxieties.

The good news is that these are all normal and common fears—most men have these as they age. In fact, many younger and middle-aged men have similar fears! But it is also important to know that most of these fears can be eliminated when the facts are known.

Throughout this book we have presented the most common facts about impotence and have given you many practical strategies for overcoming this problem. But for those men who do not know the facts, lack of knowledge about erectile dysfunction can cause unnecessary worries, which may lead to physical conditions such as hypertension (high blood pressure). High blood pressure needs medications to treat it—medications that often have impotence as a side effect. This is just one case where if you take care of the anxiety before it gets out of control, you can save yourself a lot of stress later on.

As we stated earlier, studies show that unresolved stress accounts for up to 80 percent of all diseases. Imagine how our lives would be if we could only conquer this enemy of our mind instead of letting it play fascinating tricks on us.

Even though physical and intellectual setbacks are more numerous and frequent (though by no means unavoidable) in old age, if you can learn how to control and replace fearful thoughts with positive ones, you will help yourself move beyond impotence to discover a better quality of life.

> "When my doctor first confirmed that I was impotent, I wanted to run and hide. The initial shock of hearing those words gave me great anxiety and worry.
> —Scott, investment banker, 53"

Regaining Control

Men who live with impotence for long periods of time may become withdrawn and depressed—so much so that they spend a great deal of time away from their spouses.

As time goes on, the stress of dealing with impotence can cause severe strain on the marriage, resulting in divorce or irreparable communication problems. The longer the impotence lasts, the more likely the man—and often his wife—will experience symptoms of stress.

If you are impotent, it is important to understand the problem and actively seek a solution before it becomes one more key stressor in your already stressed life. Your goal should be to find treatment that can help you return to sexual activity in your relationship without fear of erectile dysfunction. You can learn to live with this common problem—and overcome the dysfunction using medical or complementary treatments.

Just the Facts

- Stress describes the many demands and pressures that all people experience to some degree each day.
- Alcohol and drug abuse used to mask feelings of hopelessness may further hinder sexual function.
- Impotence can lead to an emotional state that includes anxiety, fear, and even depression.

PART IV

Evaluating Impotency Solutions

Chapter 11

GET THE SCOOP ON...

The specific chemicals necessary for strong erections ▪ How Viagra works to increase erections ▪ Who should take Viagra because of certain medical conditions or medications ▪ Side effects that may occur with Viagra

The Love Drug: Viagra

On March 17, 1998, the Food and Drug Administration (FDA) approved Pfizer Pharmaceuticals' impotence "cure," Viagra (sildenafil citrate). As the first oral therapy for male erectile dysfunction, the $10 apiece tiny blue diamond-shaped pills have captured everyone's attention. And, even though insurers are reimbursing only a small percentage of users, projected sales are already estimated at more than $1 billion in the first year.

Plus, Viagra has not only solved the impotence problem for millions of men, it has also forced the once taboo topic of impotence into the open. It makes sense that once you know how the male body functions, you can better understand why impotence occurs and why treatments like Viagra may work in your situation.

Understanding Erections

After years of speculation, scientists now understand how the male penile erection works. With this knowledge, the race began to develop medications to overcome erectile dysfunction.

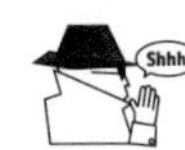

Unofficially... When the penis is fully erect, it holds about five to eight times more blood than when flaccid. The blood should remain in the erect penis until you reach an orgasm and ejaculation.

The first oral medications such as yohimbine (Yocon) have not been very effective. In fact, some studies show that yohimbine's success rate in clinical trials is only 20 percent effective, while placebos (sugar tablets) worked in 15 percent of clinical trials. Also, although yohimbine has been approved for use by the FDA, that same agency has deemed the herb "unsafe." Hoping to come up with treatments to help impotent men, scientists have developed penile injections, vacuum devices, medications inserted into the urethra, and even surgical procedures, all of which will be discussed in Chapter 12.

Sex starts in your mind

Testosterone is a major cause of your libido, the sexual drive. When the libido is working well, your brain receives erotic stimulation from your senses (touch, vision, hearing, or even imagination). Once these senses are processed, the brain sends messages to the rest of the body.

Scientists have realized that some chemicals that the body produces stimulate sexual behavior and stronger erections, while other chemicals can slow down this process.

When you are sexually aroused, your brain's messages cause stimulation of the parasympathetic nerves to the penis. This, in turn, causes the nerve endings to release specific chemicals in parts of the penis (the corpora cavernosum, two erectile bodies, see Chapter 1), which create erections.

The corpora cavernosum act like sponges in your penis. As the blood flows into these bodies, they begin to swell and the penis grows larger. When all of the spaces are filled with blood, the penis becomes stiff and rigid. The penis stays rigid because the blood-filled corpora cavernosum exert strong pressure against the penile veins, reducing the chances of blood flowing out (see Figures 11.1 and 11.2).

FIGURE 11.1: A FLACCID PENIS (TISSUE WITHOUT EXTRA BLOOD)

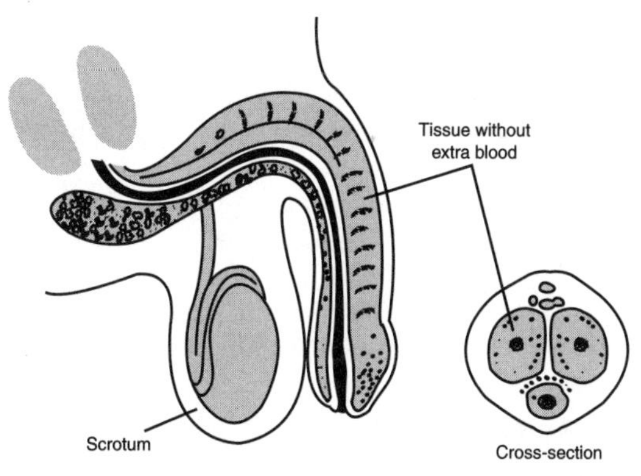

FIGURE 11.2: A NORMALLY ERECT PENIS (TISSUE FILLED WITH EXTRA BLOOD)

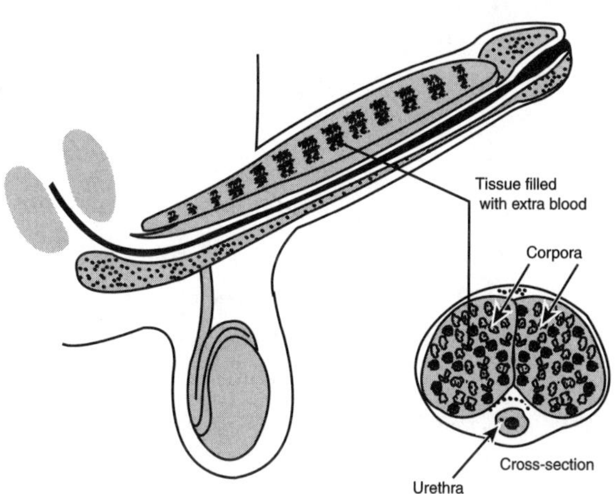

> "While men are quick to comment about their wives' hot flashes, they do not want to hear about changes their own bodies undergo at midlife. They are afraid of losing their macho image and walk around pretending nothing has changed since their early twenties. When you deny treatment for impotence, you keep from fully enjoying your life.
> —Brett, sex therapist, 51"

Nitric oxide: the erection chemical

Through comprehensive research, scientists have found that the chemical nitric oxide is especially important for erections to occur. When nitric oxide is released, an enzyme reaction produces a chemical called cyclic GMP, which causes the small arteries in the penis to dilate or become larger, allowing more blood to enter the penis. During this process there is relaxation of small involuntary muscles in the corpora cavernosum, and the veins taking blood away from the penis are narrowed so more blood enters the penis than exits. The erection is created and will remain so as long as the penis is engorged with blood or usually until after ejaculation.

Back to normal

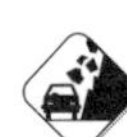

Watch Out! The FDA also warns that the sudden exertion involved in resuming sexual activity may be too risky for men with heart conditions and urges doctors to assess heart health before prescribing Viagra.

Once you experience an orgasm, the sympathetic nerve stimulation causes the small arteries to constrict, and blood flow into the penis decreases. The veins allow more blood to exit, and the erection stops until the next time your body is aroused or your penis is directly stimulated.

The Viagra/Erection Connection

Approved by the FDA in 1998, Viagra is the first oral medication to be released for treatment of erectile dysfunction.

The upside

Even though Viagra was formulated to treat impotence, you still must have sexual stimulation for it to work. In other words, you cannot take this pill and then magically have an erection. Like a normal erection, arousal must start in your mind, with direct stimulation of the penis. It works by increasing the level of the chemical cyclic GMP, which has a positive effect on erections.

A major advantage of Viagra is that it comes in an easy-to-take tablet form. This offers more discretion and convenience than other erectile dysfunction treatments.

The clinical trials on Viagra demonstrated the positive effect this pill has on sexual function in men. Test studies reveal that of the 3,000 men with erectile dysfunction who took Viagra, improvement in erections occurred in 82 percent of the 380 subjects who took 100 mg; 74 percent of the 391 who took 50 mg; and 63 percent of the 214 who took 25 mg. Twenty-four percent of the 463 test subjects who took placebo treatment also showed improvement.

Some men in the clinical trials of Viagra noticed an effect as early as 30 minutes after taking the medication. Many reported being able to get an erection for up to four hours after they took Viagra, while some men noticed improvement as late as the next day.

Men whose erectile dysfunction was caused by various maladies such as vascular disease or diabetes, or occurred as a side effect of medications, all received improvement from Viagra. Even men who had undergone prostate surgery (which can cause impotence), and those with spinal cord injuries, reported positive results from this pill.

In 532 men with erectile dysfunction who took Viagra in the privacy of their homes, those who received 100 mg had twice as many erections with treatment as opposed to times when they had no treatment. Sixty-nine percent of all attempts at sexual intercourse were successful in those who took Viagra, yet only 22 percent who took placebos told of having successful erections. Those who took Viagra had 5.9 successful attempts at intercourse per month, while those who took a placebo had 1.5. These scores approached the reports of normal men of the same age, although a reviewer did point out that the erections did not equal what normal men achieved in terms of strength and duration of erection.

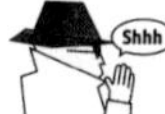

Unofficially... During Viagra's first two months of availability, about 42 percent of users were 40 to 59 years old, 12.9 percent were 60 to 64 years old, and 28.5 percent were 65 to 74 years old. Only three percent were between 20 and 39 years old.

Some researchers have found that Viagra may lower blood pressure slightly in patients who were not experiencing erectile dysfunction.

The downside

The downside of taking Viagra is that it may not work for you. In clinical trials, not all men had successful intercourse each time, and a host of men reported mild side effects. Keep in mind these side effects were not life-threatening and for the most part were simply annoying. The most common side effects were slight headache, flushing, indigestion, nasal congestion, and mild temporary visual disturbance with changes in color hue (usually blue-green) or brightness. The side effects in this study were reported by researchers to be usually very slight, lasting a few minutes to a few hours after taking the medication.

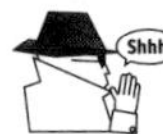

Unofficially... After taking Viagra, 16 to 30 percent of men reported having headaches, and from three to 11 percent reported vision changes. Vision may become blue-tinged and blurred due to a chemical reaction in the cells of the retina. The drug can also cause sensitivity to light. Both effects are temporary, but whether there are any long-term effects is not known.

Unlike other erectile dysfunction treatments, studies on Viagra found no priapism (a painful, prolonged erection) as a side effect. Priapism can happen with some medications that are inserted into the urethra (the tube which carries urine through the penis, and where the medication is then absorbed into the penis) or with medications that are directly injected into the penis.

Serious contraindications with nitroglycerin

Patients taking nitroglycerin, or similar nitrate-based heart medications, may experience sudden large drops in blood pressure when Viagra is also taken. This can be dangerous for patients who have heart disease or other vascular problems and can even be fatal. It is especially dangerous for patients who don't inform the doctor treating their impotence about their other medications or their heart disease. Don't risk death in order to solve your problem with impotence.

In the clinical trials before the drug was approved there were reported to be eight deaths among patients who also had serious risks for heart disease. The FDA felt Viagra itself was not to blame, and the concern was raised about the combination of nitrate-related drugs and Viagra. There were around 30 reports of deaths during the first two months after Viagra was released, including a few who died during sexual activity.

Timesaver
For more information on Viagra, including the FDA's clinical review of the studies, approval letter, and labeling, check out the Internet site: http://www.fda.gov/cder/news/viagra.htm.

However, death from sexual activity is not unheard of among heart disease patients even without the use of Viagra. This is because the physical exertion of the sexual activity, which increases the work of the heart, may bring on chest pain. Many heart patients routinely take nitroglycerin when they have chest pain from exertion, since the chest pain (angina pectoris) is caused by the heart disease. But if nitroglycerin is taken for chest pain after sex and after Viagra, the combination could be deadly.

TABLE 11.1: COMMONLY PRESCRIBED NITRATES AND MEDICATIONS THAT SHOULD NOT BE TAKEN WITH VIAGRA

Cardilate	Cartrax	Deponit (transdermal)	Dilitrate
Dilitrate SR	Duotrate	Imdur	Ismo
Iso-D	Isordil	Isotrate	Minitran Transdermal Systems
Miltrate	Miltrate 10	Monoket	Nitrek
Nitro-Bid	Nitrocine	Nitorcot	Nitrol Ointment (Appli-Kit)
Nitro-Derm	Nitrogard	Nitroglyn	Nitrolingual Spray
Nitrong	Nitropar	Nitropress	Nitrostat
Nitro-Time	Onset-5	Papavarral	Pennate
Penta Cap #1	Pentrate	Penitrol	Peritrate
Sorvide-10	Sorbitrate	Sorbitrate SR	Tetrate-30
Transderm-Nitro	Transdermal NTG	Tridil	

How to take Viagra

For most men, the usual dose is one 50 mg tablet taken about one hour before sexual activity. Viagra can also be taken from 30 minutes to four hours before sexual activity (the response may happen within 30 minutes, and the effect may last 4 hours or more in some persons). The dose can be decreased to 25 mg or increased to 100 mg if needed. For those over age 65, a starting dose of 25 mg may be sufficient. Do not take Viagra more than once each day.

Watch Out! Do not ever take Viagra if you take nitroglycerin or nitrate-related medications, including the nitrate skin patch, or if you might need to take nitroglycerin for chest pain.

Having Safe Sex Using Viagra

If you are impotent and feel that Viagra might help get your sex life back on track, there are certain steps to consider. First, keep in mind that age, diseases, anxiety, and stress all can interfere with the ability to have an erection. Impotence may be caused by:

- Diabetes, which can damage blood vessels and nerves
- Prostate cancer surgery
- Spinal injury
- Hormonal imbalances
- Alcohol and drug abuse
- Heart problems
- Blocked arteries
- Diuretics
- Cortisone drugs
- Medications
- Depression
- Emotions, such as anxiety or fear

Talk with your doctor

Since impotence may be a sign of a pre-existing medical disorder, every man who experiences erection problems should seek help from a qualified physician (family physician, internist, or urologist).

Seeing your doctor before embarking on any "treatment" for impotence will ensure a proper and potentially life-saving medical diagnosis and treatment. Once these problems are treated, your impotence may also go away. In other words, treating the initial problem may put you back in working order—without Viagra or any of the other erectile dysfunction treatments.

Many of the problems that can contribute to erectile dysfunction can also increase your chance of heart disease. These include diabetes, peripheral vascular disease in the legs, smoking, and hypertension.

If you already know you have heart disease, even if you don't take nitroglycerin or related products, talk to your doctor before taking Viagra. Be sure it's safe for you before you take any risk. Also, if you have risk factors for coronary heart disease, such as hypertension, high blood cholesterol, diabetes, or if you smoke cigarettes, talk with your doctor before taking Viagra. It may be necessary to do tests to ensure there is no underlying coronary heart disease.

Start with the lowest dosage

If your doctor has agreed that Viagra may help your erectile dysfunction, be sure to start with the lowest dose. This is either 25 mg or 50 mg.

It's important to avoid alcohol while taking Viagra, and keep in mind that a large, heavy meal may interfere with the absorption.

> "Viagra changed our marriage. My husband had been impotent for six years until his urologist suggested he try Viagra. This is a wonder drug in our estimation. —Paula, homemaker, 52"

Arousal still required

Remember, Viagra is not magic. It will not work unless you are sexually stimulated or aroused. The same type of foreplay you used to create an erection before becoming impotent is still needed to trigger the chemical response from Viagra.

A word of warning

Taking Viagra to have bigger or better erections—even though you are not impotent—is not recommended. Viagra cannot help your sexual function if you don't have erectile dysfunction. Other cautions include:

- Do not ever take Viagra if you take nitroglycerin or nitrate-related products as it may result in a severe drop in blood pressure. Deaths have been reported from this combination of medications and this warning must be adhered to.
- If you are taking erythromycin, Biaxin, ketoconazole, or itraconazole—commonly prescribed antibiotics—ask your doctor before taking Viagra. There may be a drug/drug interaction that you must be aware of and it's better to be safe than sorry.
- If you have liver or kidney disease, check with your doctor before taking Viagra. While test studies do not show a problem with liver or kidney function, only your doctor knows your situation and can advise you best.
- If you have Peyronie's disease (deviation in direction of the penis on erection), sickle cell disease, leukemia or multiple myeloma, a bleeding disorder, or retinitis pigmentosa, check with your doctor before you take Viagra.

- If you are at high risk for heart disease or stroke (you smoke cigarettes, have hypertension, high blood cholesterol, diabetes mellitus, or are overweight), talk with your doctor before you take Viagra. Clinical trials do not link these conditions to problems with Viagra, but these conditions could create problems if you over-exert yourself during the sexual act itself. Sexual activity generally involves an increase in cardiac work and myocardial oxygen demand, which for some men could be dangerous or even deadly, depending on their cardiac condition.
- Keep in mind that Viagra does not work for every man. If it does not work in your situation, see Chapter 13 for other effective treatments.
- Viagra is not approved for use in women, but studies are in progress to see how well it works.

Watch Out!
Healthcare professionals are encouraged by the FDA to report any serious adverse events that are associated with the use of Viagra. Contact the FDA's MedWatch program by phone (1-800-FDA-1088), fax (1-800-FDA-0178) or mail to FDA, HF-2, 5600 Fishers Lane, Rockville, MD 20852-9787, or to Pfizer (1-800-438-1985).

Keep talking

Keep communication open with your doctor. Do not hide any information about other medical problems or medications, and if you notice any side effects, check with your doctor before using it again.

Be sure to watch out for a host of imposter drugs, herbs, and other treatments. Some of these drugs may look or sound like Viagra, so be aware.

Knowing When NOT to Use Viagra

The FDA, in conjunction with Pfizer Pharmaceuticals, has identified specific situations in which taking Viagra could be extremely dangerous, even to the point of causing death.

One such contradindication for taking Viagra is while you are taking an organic nitrate. Unfortunately, there are several ways this may be given to

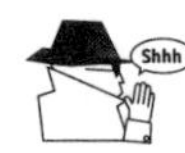

Unofficially... Experts believe that the problem of impotence is much more widespread than the earlier estimates of 30 million men. The new comprehensive Massachusetts Male Health Study found about 52 percent of men 40 to 70 experience some degree of impotence.

you—without your knowledge. If nitroglycerin or isosorbide mononitrate is taken when Viagra is in your system, it can result in large and sudden drops in systemic blood pressure. A list of commonly prescribed short- and long-acting nitrates is given in Table 11.1 (above).

Viagra and angina

There are situations where men, especially those who become sexually active after abstaining for a period of time, with a history of angina might take Viagra and a nitrate. The aerobic activity of having sex is enough to precipitate an anginal attack. The treatment for this? Nitroglycerin—a dangerous and perhaps deadly combination if Viagra is in your system.

If the nitroglycerin is taken while Viagra is in the body, you could become acutely hypotensive, that is, experience a rapid drop in blood pressure. This great drop in blood pressure could have no symptoms at all or bring on the following symptoms:

- Dizziness
- Light-headedness
- Fainting (in severe cases)

With hypotension, you could end up in an ambulance or an emergency room.

Viagra and first-time angina

Then there's the man with no history of angina who takes Viagra, engages in sexual activity, and experiences his first anginal episode. Such a patient could be brought to an emergency room while still having chest pain, where a short-acting nitrate may routinely be administered to treat this. If the emergency room doctor is not aware of the potential interaction described above, and does not specifically question the patient about Viagra, he may administer nitroglycerin—with potentially deadly results.

Another possible scenario would be if you called 911 because you had chest pain and a team of paramedics or EMTs responded to this call. In some cities, these emergency personnel are allowed to immediately give a short-acting nitrate on the scene or in the ambulance. If this happens while Viagra is still in your system, the consequences could be serious, even deadly.

Viagra and inhaled nitrates

Illegal recreational inhaled nitrates, such as amyl nitrate and butyl nitrate, can cause a serious reaction when combined with Viagra. These inhaled nitrates, called "poppers," are often used as an aphrodisiac.

Viagra and the opposite sex

Although Viagra is only FDA-approved for the treatment of male erectile dysfunction, we are aware that women have started taking it, either on their own or via an off-label prescription from a physician. Therefore, although the scenarios described above would be more likely to occur in men, if such off-label use continues, they could also occur in women.

“ I make some older men with a history of heart disease have a stress test before prescribing Viagra. Sometimes the added exertion of having sex—after years of abstaining—is enough to cause heart problems. —Steven, cardiologist, 46

Just the Facts

- In some clinical trials, more than 80 percent of men trying Viagra experienced erections.
- Viagra works by increasing the level of the chemical *cyclic GMP, nitric oxide,* which has a positive effect on erections.
- Viagra should never be taken by anyone who takes nitroglycerin, as the results could be deadly.

Chapter 12

GET THE SCOOP ON...

Other impotence treatments that may be more effective than Viagra ▪ Why injectable therapy may cause scarring ▪ How needleless medication is effective and easy to use ▪ Types of surgical implants that may work for you

Prostheses, Vacuums, and Other Devices

In the midst of all the media hoopla, the miracle impotence drug Viagra has done a great service for all men with erectile dysfunction. Why? Because today the subject of erectile dysfunction is now commonly discussed. You hear about it daily on the news. It is the topic of conversation at parties and is no longer hiding in secrecy, destroying the lives of millions of men and women.

While many men can use Viagra with great success, what happens to those who, for various reasons, cannot take this medication? What about those men who suffer from impotence but cannot afford Viagra or the ones who cannot take it because they also take nitroglycerin? Are there other viable solutions to correct erectile dysfunction?

The good news is that treatments for impotence are varied and many; every man with erectile dysfunction can once again have a quality sexual life.

A Shot of Hope

Perhaps it sounds a little gruesome at first, but you'll find that injections of medications into the penis do work. In fact, in about 90 percent of all cases, injection therapy is successful for ending erectile dysfunction.

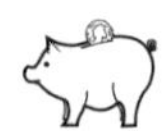

Moneysaver Studies show that 78 percent of patients using Vivus, Inc.'s Muse system were reimbursed by insurance companies, while 68 percent of patients using Pharmacia & Upjohn, Inc.'s Caverject product were reimbursed. Muse and Caverject use a different active ingredient than Viagra.

How it works

The idea is that an injection into the erection chambers of the penis puts the drug exactly where it is needed to work.

After the medication is injected (see Figure 12.1), the small arteries in the penis open wider and blood flow increases. The veins that control blood flow out of the penis also constrict, thus allowing the penis to become engorged and an erection to occur.

The upside

Researchers have found injectable treatments to be one of the most effective for ending impotence. The medication is injected before sexual activity, and the erection usually develops within about 10 to 15 minutes, and lasts for around two hours.

Injections naturally make some people nervous or squeamish; perhaps more so given the location of this injection. There is nothing to fear. The procedure is simple, but it is important to know how to correctly inject the medication for the best effect. Your doctor will show you the actual technique, which is easy to learn. It's important that the injection be in the exact area of one side of the penis.

If you choose to try injections to stop impotence, you need to have regular check-ups and follow-ups with your urologist to check for side effects. Your doctor will test varying doses of medication to see which ones produce the best effect in your case.

The downside

It's important to monitor the length of time your penis stays erect to prevent prolonged erections. Prolonged erections, which last for hours, are less common than with other medications used for impotence, but they can happen. It is important when you use injection treatments that you know what to do if a prolonged (more than four hours) or painful erection occurs. Prolonged erections should be treated seriously as an emergency. You should already know from your doctor's instructions what to do and what phone number to call.

Watch Out!
Do not ever use injection therapy until your doctor ensures you can do it safely!

FIGURE 12.1: INJECTION TREATMENT FOR IMPOTENCE

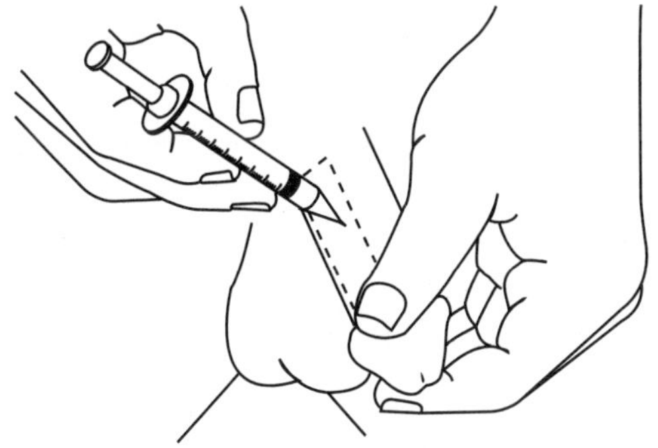

It may take a few visits to your doctor to find the correct dosage.

One frequent side effect of injection treatment is a thickening of the tissues in the penis, which does, however, often diminish after treatments are stopped. Burning during injections or painful erections are more common with this treatment and are the most common reason for trying other types of treatment.

Injection therapy is also expensive, costing twice as much as Viagra per treatment (about $20 per injection).

What's available

Caverject or Edex (alprostadil is the generic name) is one of a group of medications called prostaglandins (prostaglandin E) which widens the small arteries in the penis, narrows the veins leading away from the penis, and increases the chance of a successful erection. The success rate with Caverject or Edex averages over 90 percent for erections.

Researchers have found a combination of the medications papaverine and phentolamine to have a high rate of success, with an average success rate of more than 70 percent. Prolonged erection is the most common side effect, though most patients experience no side effects. Thickening or scarring is uncommon, but can happen. Regular check-ups with your urologist can help minimize side effects. Since this treatment is directed at the arteries, it may not work as well in cases of severe arterial blockage. Papaverine (this is the generic name) has been widely used by urologists, with an average success rate of more than 50 percent. As with other injected medications, prolonged erection is possible, as is thickening of the penis from scarring at the injection site. Both of these side effects are, however, uncommon. Follow up with your doctor to prevent and manage these effects. This treatment is also less effective in persons who have severe arterial disease with limited blood flow in the arteries to the penis.

Newer medications can be used alone or in combination. Invicorp is a ready-filled auto-injector that many persons may find easier to use. Invicorp combines VIP (vasoactive intestinal polypeptide) with phentolamine and has been reported to have an almost 70-percent success rate in men for whom other injections had not been successful.

Pump It Up

A vacuum constriction device requires no injection or other medication and is effective in most cases of erectile dysfunction. The one-time cost for this device is about $400 to $500.

How it works

A vacuum constriction device uses a plastic cylinder, a constriction ring, and a pump, which can be manual or battery operated (see Figure 12.2).

FIGURE 12.2: A VACUUM CONSTRICTION DEVICE TO TREAT IMPOTENCE

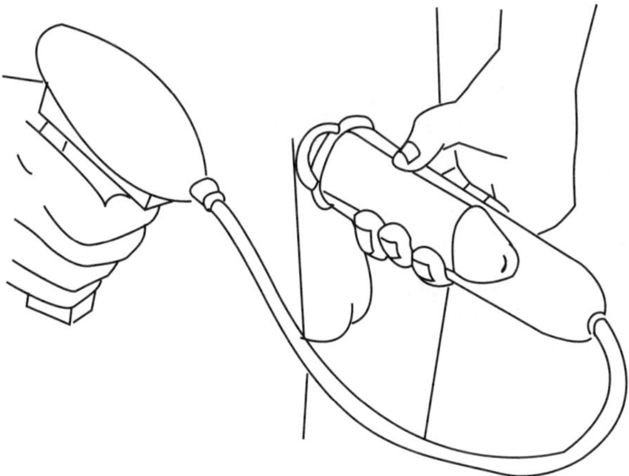

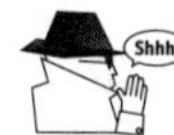

Unofficially... The success rate for men using vacuum constriction devices is 90 percent or better.

The penis is inserted into the open end of the cylinder, which is clear plastic. The device is held against the abdominal wall to keep an airtight seal. The pump is then used to remove air from the cylinder. This negative pressure draws blood into the penis and creates an erection. When the erection is as desired, with the cylinder still in place, the constriction ring at the open end of the cylinder is moved off the cylinder to the base of the penis. The ring is worn during intercourse. This compresses

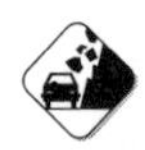

Watch Out! If you take a blood thinner such as Coumadin (warfarin) you should check with your doctor before using a vacuum device, although its use is usually still possible. If you have sickle cell anemia or priapism (prolonged erections) you should ask your doctor before you use the device.

the veins and keeps more blood in the penis to help maintain the erection. It usually takes about two to three minutes to create an erection, and the ring can be left on for 30 minutes. The erection often is maintained after orgasm. The ring should be removed after 30 minutes to avoid complications.

The upside

The greatest benefit for the vacuum constriction device is that most men will find that it helps them to achieve successful erections. Plus, because it is not a medication, there are no side effects. Although use of the tension ring creates some discomfort, this is not usually a major, limiting problem. The need to use the device can interfere with sexual activity, but this is usually not a big problem once the couple becomes used to the device, especially since the success rate is high.

In scientific studies, more than 80 percent of patients with a history of prostate surgery said they achieved good erections with the application of vacuum therapy. About 22 percent said that after three months of using vacuum therapy, they were able to achieve spontaneous erections at least some of the time.

The downside

The device may cause bruises on the penis, especially if the pressure is held too long or if the vacuum is created too rapidly. This can usually be avoided by watching through the clear plastic. Newer models have devices that can help prevent excessive negative pressure in the cylinder.

Most side effects become less bothersome after the device is used more than a few times, and bruises can usually be minimized with experience.

Needleless Medicines May Solve Your Problem

The medicated urethral system for erection (MUSE) uses alprostadil, the same prostaglandin drug discussed earlier, to achieve an erection. This is an insertable treatment in which the drug is directly inserted into the urethra, the tube in the penis that leads from the bladder. The medication is then absorbed through the lining of the urethra.

How it works

It is recommended that you urinate first, then shake the penis to remove excess urine. Check to see that the medication pellet is at the end of the applicator, and gently stretch the penis to make it straight (this also makes the urethra straighter).

Insert the pellet of medication on the applicator into the opening of the urethra (see Figure 12.3). Then gently push down the button on the top of the applicator until it stops and hold for about five seconds. Gently move the applicator from side to side to allow the pellet of medication to separate in the urethra. Remove the applicator while keeping the penis upright, and extend the penis to its full length and gently roll it between your hands for 10 seconds. You need to sit, walk, or stand for about 10 minutes while the erection develops. The erection should last 30 to 60 minutes.

The upside

Studies have shown about 70 percent of patients achieved successful erection using this insertable medication, and it was effective in patients with various types of erectile dysfunction. One study showed about a 60-percent success rate in diabetic men with erectile dysfunction.

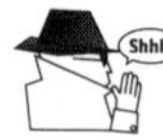

Unofficially... The new American Urological Association (AUA) guidelines state that vacuum therapy, injection therapy, and surgically implanted penile prostheses are all safe and effective treatments for erectile dysfunction. This organization urges physicians to fully inform patients (and partners) in an unbiased manner about the benefits and potential complications of each of these three treatments.

FIGURE 12.3: INSERTABLE MEDICATION HAS A HIGH SUCCESS RATE

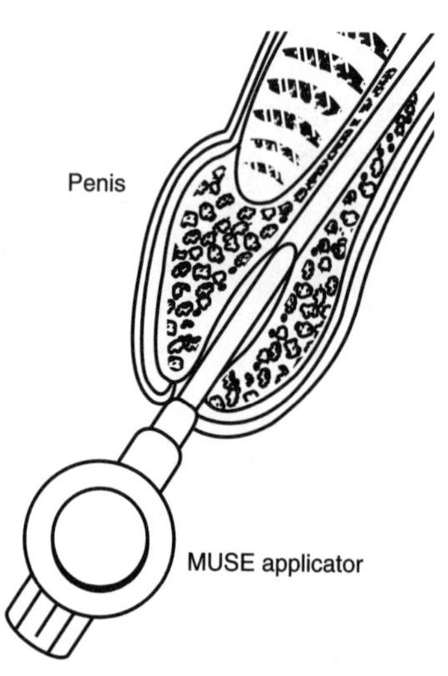

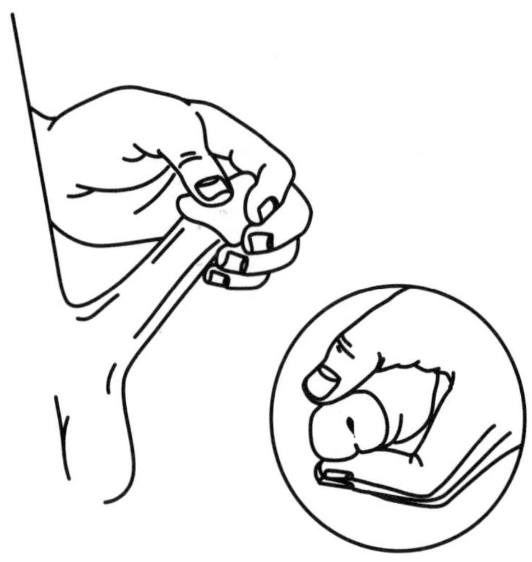

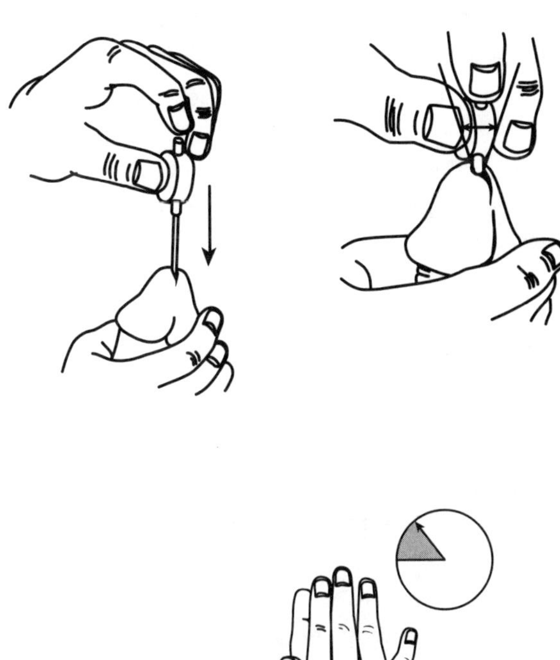

The downside

The most common side effect is pain in the penis, which is usually mild. Dizziness is an occasional, but uncommon, side effect.

If you have sickle cell trait, sickle cell disease, or a blood disorder, ask your doctor before you use MUSE.

Treatments for Venous Leakage

As discussed earlier, complete erection depends on an increase in blood flow to the penis and narrowing of the veins near the surface that take blood away from the penis. Erectile dysfunction can happen if there is not enough blood flowing into the penis, or if the veins do not remain sufficiently narrowed to maintain an erection. If the small muscles in this area do not relax, blood will flow out of the penis instead of being trapped, and there is a good chance that the erection will not be maintained.

How it works

In these cases, treatment options can include a latex band to create enough constriction to direct blood flow away from the penis, which can maintain the erection. The latex rubber loop, which the user can easily control to adjust the amount of compression, is stretched and placed around the penis at the base (see Figure 12.4).

One end of the latex band is pulled away from the penis until the band is snug around the base. The tension of the latex band can be increased or lessened to have the desired effect on the erection, which should be the least tension needed to maintain the erection. After use, it is loosened and removed. Like the vacuum device, this method requires no injections or medications that might have side effects.

The downside

Don't use this device if you have sickle cell trait or anemia, a deformity of the penis, leukemia, multiple myeloma, or other conditions that cause abnormal blood clotting. Do not maintain tension for more than 30 minutes at one time, and wait at least 60 minutes between uses. Excessive or too frequent use can cause bruising of the penis. It should not be used when you are under the influence of alcohol or sedatives (so you don't fall asleep with tension on the penis). Pain or redness of the penis or prolonged erection can occur. As with other treatments, if an erection lasts longer than four hours, treat it as an emergency and call your doctor.

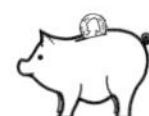

Moneysaver
Yohimbine tablets cost about $40 a month. Before you spend money, however, keep in mind that the success rate is low—only 20 percent in case studies (a sugar tablet works in 15 percent of cases).

Other Alternatives to Treat Impotence

Viagra is the major oral treatment because it is convenient and has a good success rate (see Chapter 11). In fact, no treatment has exhibited the dramatic results of Viagra.

Yohimbine works for some

As will be discussed in Chapter 13, yohimbine is available over the counter in many areas. It is often one of the first medications tried once the evaluation for erectile dysfunction is made. Some studies find it has some beneficial effect in cases of psychological erectile dysfunction, especially to overcome performance anxiety. Yet other studies have found no real benefit in patients with physical causes of erectile dysfunction. Some users notice anxiety, increased pulse rate, or headache.

Yohimbine is taken three times a day for four to six weeks initially. Men with hypertension or ulcers should discuss this with their doctor before taking this medication.

Vasomax (phentolamine) is available

In recent studies, some patients with erectile dysfunction benefited from taking oral doses of Vasomax (phentolamine). Over half of patients in one study were able to have an erection adequate for intercourse 75 percent of the time.

Lotions and patches hold hope for the future

Almost as convenient as a pill would be an effective lotion or patch that could produce erections. At this time, several are under development. Some are using one of the prostaglandin drugs discussed earlier.

It is likely that there will soon be choices available that may help erections either alone or in combination with another treatment.

Arterial surgery for erectile dysfunction

While surgical treatment is uncommon, men who have certain types of arterial blockage and cannot use other treatments may need to turn to surgery to cure their erectile dysfunction. This is especially useful in young men after injuries to the pelvis or nearby areas. It is not very useful for those usually older men who have more widespread artery blockage from atherosclerosis. The success of this operation depends on the individual situation. Your urologist can give you the best advice in your own case.

When to opt for a penile prosthesis

After the failure of other treatments, or after other treatments can no longer be tolerated, as a last resort penile prosthesis will allow the return of sexual activity.

Some types of prostheses contain two rods that are placed in the corpora cavernosum. The rods are permanent and the length of the penis remains the same, so it may be noticeable at times. Others are more flexible and may be preferred by many patients.

Some prostheses are inflatable, which means inflation of the penis for an erection is done by squeezing the penis, then bending it after sexual activity to release the contained fluid (see Figure 12.5). Other available prostheses contain two or three pieces—each having certain advantages and disadvantages. Talk with your urologist if you are considering this possibility.

FIGURE 12.5 IMPLANT THERAPY IS EFFECTIVE

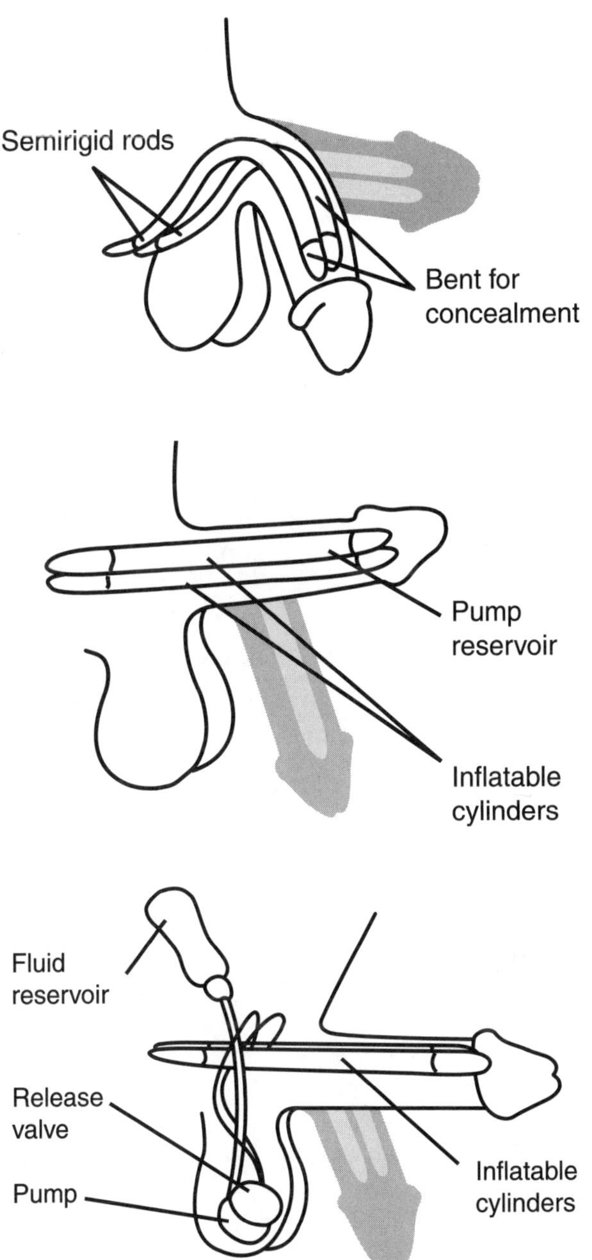

Watch Out! Because of side effects, those with prostate cancer, liver disease, heart disease, or other medical problems should not use testosterone without their doctor's advice. Also, testosterone treatments can worsen sleep apnea, aggravate prostate disease, cause blood changes, and increase the risk of stroke.

Keep in mind that this type of surgery does not change other activities such as orgasm or urination. It is usually out-patient surgery, and studies reveal that more than 90 percent of patients are satisfied. If the implant fails, then an operation is usually needed to fix the problem.

Hormone treatments

As discussed earlier, an uncommon cause of erectile dysfunction is a low level of testosterone. A low testosterone level more commonly affects sexual desire, the libido, but can occasionally also limit erections. Treatment consists of regular doses of testosterone to raise the level of the hormone. This may restore libido and erection if deficiency is the problem. It may also improve the general sense of well-being.

Just the Facts

- In almost every situation, there are many safe and effective alternatives for the treatment of impotence.
- While the vacuum erection device requires an initial cost of about $400 to $500, this is a one-time payment.
- With injection therapy, the patient injects medication into the side of the penis before intercourse.

Chapter 13

GET THE SCOOP ON...

How alternative medicines may help stress-related impotence ▪ Which herbs are commonly used to stop erectile dysfunction ▪ Certain homeopathic remedies that might help stop impotence ▪ How mind/body interplay can help you de-stress and enjoy relaxed sex

Choosing Alternative Therapies

Because impotence is often related to such lifestyle influences as too much stress, anxiety, or even exhaustion from overwork, alternative or complementary therapies may be attractive to you. Alternative medicine, also called "complementary" or "unconventional" medicine, views the mind and body as an integrated system, meaning they influence each other. This method of treatment depends on your total involvement with staying well or self-care.

In the past three decades, alternative medicine has soared in popularity and touts a wide range of non-standard approaches to personal health and healing. Some, like yoga and herbal treatments, are steeped in ancient Asian traditions; others, like art, dance, or music therapy. are strictly New Age; all have proponents from every walk of life who vouch for their healing powers.

The skyrocketing use of complementary medicine represents a growing dissatisfaction with conventional or allopathic healthcare.

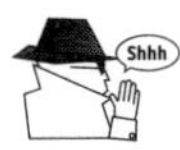

Unofficially... Allopaths, or conventional medical doctors, focus upon defining disease based on measurable symptoms and eliminating those signs; alternative therapists treat the whole person—body, mind, and spirit—with the focus on staying balanced and well.

Although many alternative healers do not have medical degrees and are not recognized by the American Medical Association (AMA), more and more people are turning to alternative medicine because the solutions are appealing, and they offer hope. Especially with the soaring costs of health care, alternative treatments, which range from herbal supplements to meditation, are relatively affordable, easily accessible, and allow you to participate actively in key decisions about your health.

Less Stress Means Stronger Erections

As you recall, stress is a leading cause of impotence. But how can mind/body therapies balance your life, helping you regain control of your life, while also ending your impotence?

Focusing on the mind/body connection

To begin with, alternative therapies are based on the premise that the mind and body are interconnected to an extent far surpassing previous assumptions, and physical health and emotional well-being are closely linked. For example, scientific tests demonstate that stress can literally wreck your health. In today's pressured society, chronic stress can persist for days, weeks, or even months, tearing at your mind, body, and spirit.

While each man is different, many believe that alternative therapies can put them back in control, and self-efficacy or control is essential for wellness—and for a good erection. Remember how just the "fear" of erectile dysfunction may cause it to occur? Feeling that you are in control of your environment and your body will also help you have better control during sex.

A holistic approach

Instead of prescribing an expensive pharmaceutical as the cure for an illness, alternative practitioners focus on the ideas of natural medicine, holism, and wellness. In fact, most alternative practitioners take into account all parts of the person, not just the part that has the symptom.

To help you understand how alternative medicine really works, think back to the last time you had an excruciating headache. What treatment finally worked to relieve your pain? If you go to a conventional medical doctor with headache as your symptom, he may run some laboratory tests, then give you a prescription pain reliever or antibiotic for infection. If you see a holistic practitioner with headache as your symptom, she may review your history, ask questions about your lifestyle, then prescribe various treatments that would work together to reconnect the mind and body and help you to do the following:

- Reduce your tension with biofeedback.
- Decrease pain with feverfew, an herb that has been found to help with migraine pain.
- Eliminate toxins from your body by increasing fluids and clear liquids.
- Visualize being "pain free" using guided imagery and imagination.
- Increase healing sleep with hydrotherapy (a warm bath).
- Strengthen the immune system using nutritional supplements.

Bright Idea
Eating certain foods may have an amorous effect on the body. For example, chocolate contains phenylethylamine (PEA), a chemical the body produces when we are in love, and may give the libido a lift. Likewise, studies show that the smell of pumpkin pie and doughnuts can arouse sexual desires in men.

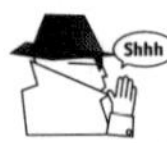

Unofficially... In terms of lost hours due to absenteeism, reduced productivity, and workers' compensation benefits, stress costs American industry more than $300 billion annually. More importantly, stress can make us ill. At least four in 10 of all adults suffer adverse health effects from stress and as many as nine in 10 of all visits to doctors' offices are for stress-related complaints, according to the American Psychological Association.

Would fewer drugs mean stronger erections?

Proponents of alternative treatments claim that these non-drug (or complementary) interventions may allow you to take less medication, have fewer laboratory tests and surgeries, and actively participate in self-care. In this light, if you suffer with hypertension caused by being overweight and overly stressed, turning to complementary treatments to reduce your weight and your stress levels may lower your blood pressure. Your medical doctor could then see that you are in control of your health (and blood pressure) and allow you to take less medication. Reducing the medication may be just the trigger you need to boost strength in erections.

Find Help with Mind/Body Interventions

While severe emotional stress can cause your body to fail you (impotence!), there are many ways to reestablish harmony.

Without question, the chemicals produced during moderate exercise can be extremely beneficial in terms of enhancing blood flow in the abdomen. Regular aerobic and strengthening exercises are very effective ways to train your body to deal with stress. And, of course, we've already mentioned the importance of nutrition to your health. When it comes to virility, we are indeed what we eat.

One of the most effective interventions, which costs very little money yet may help you overcome impotence, is social support. For example, loneliness may be as much a risk factor for disease as having high cholesterol or smoking cigarettes. It is well documented that people who are happily married and/or have large networks of friends not only have greater life expectancies compared with those people who do not, but they also have fewer incidences of just about all types of disease.

Plus, social support does not have to be restricted to relationships with other people. You might form emotional attachments with your animals. This is every bit as strong as the attachment between a parent and a child. Countless papers published in the area of animal/human bonding demonstrate the health benefits of this type of interaction. Even having a plant can be beneficial. This was revealed in a study conducted at Yale University by Dr. Judy Rhodin, who found that when people had a plant present in their room they had speedier recoveries compared with people who did not. The common denominator among all these studies is the word responsibility—responsibility for a loved one, for a pet, and even a plant. Taking this idea one step further, we believe that accepting responsibility for your personal health is by itself a behavioral intervention that may help you overcome impotence.

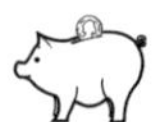

Moneysaver
Many mind/body therapies can be learned by reading how-to books or watching an instructional video. Before you spend a great deal of money, try to teach yourself methods of relaxation and stress reduction.

Mental Aerobics Work to De-Stress the Body

Psychoneuroimmunology (PNI) is the field that examines the interplay between the mind and body. Scientists know that our thoughts and feelings influence the body through the nervous and circulatory systems. These are the pathways of communication between the brain and the rest of the body. When the body is exposed to a threatening situation, we prepare for confrontation and react with the "fight or flight" response.

While we have no control over life's stressors, there are a host of mind/body therapies we can use to lessen the impact of stress. Research has shown that a healthy mind can greatly improve the functioning of our immune system, and mind/body therapies can help switch your body into a calmer mode. It makes sense that if your brain is calm, the connection between the brain and the penis will be smooth and effective—no fears, worries, or anxieties to create glitches resulting in impotence.

Bright Idea
Ask your alternative practitioner about an ayurvedic herb, Withania somnifera, or "ashwaganda" (Indian name). This herb is used for sexual deficiency in men and comes in capsules. Be sure to follow package recommendations for dosage.

Autogenics

This method of "cueing" yourself to calm down and relax is easy to perform and can be done anywhere. Because the brain only needs a few reminders to calm down, autogenics teaches you to concentrate on raising the temperature of your hands and feet. Proponents claim that autogenics will give your heart a break from pumping so hard, open blood vessels, reduce breathing rate and pulse, and lower blood pressure. With autogenics, you sit quietly, and put your left hand in your lap, palm up. Lay your right palm on top of it, and clasp your fingers together. Concentrating on the feeling in your hands, "mindfully" work to raise the temperature of your hands for 10 minutes, then do the same with your feet. Counselors claim that if this is done correctly, you will feel "the heat" rise in your hands and feet.

Deep Abdominal Breathing

Many people breathe from their chest, taking shallow, rapid breaths, but this type of breathing only hinders relaxation. Taking slow, deep "abdominal" breaths not only oxygenates the brain, it helps to end the stress cycle and enables your heart rate and blood pressure to return to normal. The brain makes its own morphine-like pain relievers, called endorphins and enkephalins that are associated with a happy, positive feeling. These hormones can help relay "stop-pain" messages. During deep abdominal breathing, you will add oxygen to the blood and cause your body to release endorphins, while decreasing the release of stress hormones.

Laughter Therapy

Can a laugh a day keep the doctor away? Maybe, according to many researchers. Think about it—while the findings are disheartening, it may come as no surprise that the average adult only laughs about 17 times a day, while a six-year-old laughs as many as 300 times. Laughter helps to relieve anxiety, decreases stress-producing hormones, and increases immune system activity. In fact, many doctors are now prescribing "humor therapy" for chronically ill patients.

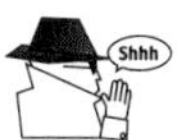

Unofficially... Some people who meditate only occasionally have opposite reactions such as increased anxiety or fear during the session. Researchers believe that these feelings may be responses to the sensation of being totally relaxed and uninhibited.

Meditation

Meditation is recognized as a viable way to lower blood pressure, alleviate insomnia, and reduce chronic pain. This stress releaser seeks to integrate the mind, body, and spirit through intentionally focusing on the silent repetition of a focus word ("love"), sound ("om"), phrase ("peace heals"), or prayer ("thank you, God"). When other thoughts intrude, continue to *mindfully* chant while facilitating the relaxation response. As a cure for impotence, this technique can guide you beyond the negative thoughts and agitations of the busy mind and allow you to become "unstuck" from your fear of not being able to "perform like a man."

Mindfulness is a traditional Buddhist approach to meditation and allows your mind to be full of whatever you are doing at that moment, whether dancing, gardening, writing, or listening to music. Intense focus is the key to mindfulness, as well as the ability to keep negative thoughts from intruding on the moment.

> "After suffering with impotence for almost a decade, I finally turned to a therapist who taught me how to relax. Using the relaxation response, music therapy, and deep abdominal breathing, I can stay focused throughout the day yet am totally free to enjoy my relationship with my wife at night.
> —Kenneth, 55, attorney"

Music Therapy

If you feel uptight after a hard day at work, keep the music playing. This form of mind/body therapy can help treat neurological, mental, or behavioral disorders such as developmental and learning disabilities, Alzheimer's disease, and other aging-related problems, brain injuries, and acute and chronic pain. Even surgeons report performing better when they could select the music played in the operating room. Composer and researcher Steven Halpern says that certain musical forms can transport the listener's brain into the alpha wave, a state of relaxation much like meditation.

Progressive Muscle Relaxation

Also known as deep muscle relaxation, this mind/body exercise involves concentrating on different muscle groups as you contract, then relax all of the major muscle groups in the body, beginning with head, neck, arms, chest, back, stomach, pelvis, legs, and feet. To do this exercise, focus on each set of muscles, tense those muscles to the count of 10, then release to the count of 10. Along with progressive muscle relaxation, it is important to perform the deep abdominal breathing, breathing in while tensing the muscles, and exhaling while relaxing them.

Relaxation Response

Achieving relaxation through the relaxation response is important in helping you reduce emotional stress. This is done by developing an inner quiet and peacefulness, a calming of negative thoughts and worries, and a mental focus away from the cares of the world. Relaxation can potentially reduce physical strain and emotional, negative thoughts—and increase your ability to self-manage stress. Each of these has a positive effect on your ability to perform sexually. And it's easy to learn.

1. Set aside a period of about 20 minutes that you can devote to relaxation practice.
2. Remove outside distractions that can disrupt your concentration: turn off the radio, the television, even the ringer on the telephone, if need be.
3. Lie flat on a bed or floor, or recline comfortably so that your whole body is supported, relieving as much tension or tightness in your muscles as you can. You can use a pillow or cushion under your head if this helps.
4. During the 20-minute period, remain as still as possible; try to focus your thoughts as much as possible on the immediate moment, and eliminate any outside thoughts which may compete for your attention.
5. As you go through these steps, in your own way try to imagine that every muscle in your body is now becoming loose, relaxed, and free of any excess tension. Picture all of the muscles in your body beginning to unwind; imagine them beginning to go loose and limp.
6. Concentrate on making your breathing even. As you exhale, picture your muscles becoming even more relaxed, as if you somehow breathe the tension away. At the end of 20 minutes, take a few moments to study and focus on the feelings and sensations you have been able to achieve. Notice whether areas that felt tight and tense at first now feel more loose and relaxed, and whether any areas of tension or tightness remain.

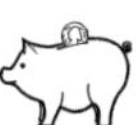

Moneysaver
Before you spend money on anti-anxiety medications, try music first. Researchers claim that listening to one half-hour of classical music produces the same effect as 10 mg of Valium—and music therapy does not have impotence as a side effect!

> "The doctor of the future will give no medicine but will interest his patient in the care of the human frame, in diet, and in the cause and prevention of disease.
> —Thomas Edison"

Visualization

Visualization (or guided imagery) is a stress-release activity that you can do wherever you are, any time of the day or night. Imagery is a flow of thoughts you can see, hear, feel, smell, or taste or an inner representation of your experiences or fantasies. This is one way your mind codes, stores, and expresses information. Imagery is also the language of emotions and the deeper self. Using visualization or imagery, you can allow your imagination to take over as you focus on your senses to create a desired state of relaxation in your mind.

1. Find a place where you can be comfortable, and allow about 15 minutes for this exercise. Sit or lie down, close your eyes, and take several deep breaths.

2. Imagine a relaxing place—somewhere you have been before so it can be visualized in your mind. This might be sitting on the seashore at sunset or sunrise, a mountain cabin next to a babbling brook, or floating on a raft in the lake on a sunny day.

3. Continue to breathe slowly and keep this image in your mind. As you explore your mental picture of your relaxing spot, imagine all the stress, worries, and tension leaving your body. Feel the temperature of your special place. See the colors and hear the sounds surrounding you. Smell the freshness of the air. Touch the gentleness of the moment. Take in all the sensory details of your relaxing place and continue to de-stress.

4. After about 15 minutes, slowly open your eyes and acclimate yourself to the surroundings in the room. Stretch your arms and legs; gently move

your head from side to side and feel the tension release. Carry the calm feeling you now have with you through the day.

- The Upside: You might see benefits from mind/body tools within minutes of doing them. For example, deep abdominal breathing actually alters your psychological state, making a painful moment diminish in intensity. Think about how your respiration quickens when you are fearful or in great pain. Then consider how taking a deep, slow breath brings an immediate calming effect, reducing both stress and levels of pain.
- The Downside: Alternative therapies are not a magic cure-all for serious health problems. If you are extremely stressed and experience such symptoms as rapid pulse or increased blood pressure, call your medical doctor for treatment.

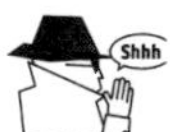

Unofficially... At this time the National Institute on Aging (NIA) is in the midst of a program to evaluate hormone therapy as a way to improve quality of life for the elderly.

Be Discerning with Alternative Therapies

Some men have found relief from impotence with herbal therapies or homeopathy. Others have turned to natural supplements (DHEA and melatonin) that are available at any health food store. But the question remains, can these really help you overcome erectile dysfunction? Perhaps, more importantly, are these supplements safe?

Whatever method you try to cure impotence, it's very important to protect yourself from media hype. Never take a "miracle" cure unless you have thoroughly read the literature and discussed it with your doctor. Most of the time if it sounds too good to be true, it is.

Yohimbine works for some

Yohimbine is an oral medication that has been taken for years by men around the world and is approved by the FDA. It is available over the counter in many areas. If you are diagnosed with erectile dysfunction, your doctor may suggest yohimbine.

- The Upside: It heightens potency by increasing blood flow to the penis. One study in California found that this herb was especially effective for treating impotence in men with diabetes and heart disease. Some studies find it has some beneficial effect in cases of psychological erectile dysfunction.
- The Downside: Other studies have found no real benefit in patients with physical causes of erectile dysfunction. Furthermore, yohimbine does increase the body's production of the adrenal hormone norepinephrine, and some users notice anxiety, increased pulse rate, or headache, which could make this unsafe for those with hypertension.

Studies affirm ginkgo biloba

Ginkgo biloba is a popular herbal treatment for impotence and has been found to relax and open up blood vessels. This may help increase male sexual performance.

- The Upside: In one German study, 20 impotent men took an 80-milligram capsule of the herb ginkgo biloba three times a day. After nine months, all were able to have spontaneous erections.
- The Downside: May cause nausea, diarrhea, stomach upset, and vomiting if larger doses are taken.

Saw palmetto for a healthy prostate

Saw palmetto has become a common herbal treatment for benign prostatic hypertrophy, or enlarged prostate, and works by relieving the main symptom of frequent urination. It is available over the counter at most grocery or drug stores and can be taken as capsules, a tincture, and fresh or dried berries.

- The Upside: Studies confirm that when taken regularly, this herbal treatment for enlarged prostate may help. It also does not appear to have the dangerous side effects that other prostate medications do.
- The Downside: Make sure you have regular prostate specific antigen (PSA) tests. Saw palmetto may help enlarged prostate, but prostate cancer will need quick medical attention.

Bright Idea
If you are taking saw palmetto, an herb said to promote prostate health, take time to tell your healthcare professional. The results of a PSA test (prostate-specific antigen test) could be affected.

Use caution with DHEA

Both men and women produce dehydroepiandrosterone (DHEA) in their adrenal glands, and men at a slightly higher level. It floods the body during youth, then dwindles as we age.

- The Upside: This anti-aging hormone is sometimes called the mother hormone because the body converts it into estrogen and testosterone. DHEA raises sex hormones and is said to make you "feel younger and sexy."
- The Downside: Researchers are quick to point out, it might also increase your chances of developing prostate cancer, or other types of cancer.

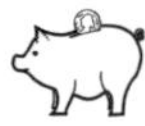

Moneysaver
Don't waste your money on a bargain; cheaper brands may have no effect at all. When buying herbal supplements, look for standardized brands. Since plants can vary significantly in their potency, the chances are greater that you will get what you pay for if you buy a brand labeled "standardized."

Weighing the benefits of melatonin

Melatonin is yet another popular hormone that can be purchased at any pharmacy or natural food store. It is produced in the pea-sized pineal gland in the center of the brain and regulates the body's circadium rhythms (daily rhythms such as your sleep/wake cycle).

- The Upside: May help improve your sleep and prevent cancer by protecting the body from free radicals. If you feel rested, this may help you perform sexually.
- The Downside: It is unregulated, untested, and may cause depression in some people.

Be discerning with herbs

Because each herb has a different property and purpose, you need to read the label or ask a practitioner for proper dosages. It is advisable to buy herbal supplements from a reliable company and to make sure they have been standardized. This means the manufacturer has performed an analytical test to measure the amount of key ingredients in the batch. Also, whole herbs that are either organic or grown in the wild have the best chances of being safe. Don't forget that dosing is not exact with herbs, and the potency can vary.

The bottom line is that many substances labeled as "natural" can also be strong medicines. Most herbal products sold in the United States are not standardized, which means that determining the exact amounts of ingredients can be difficult or impossible. Herbal preparations can affect your response to prescribed medication or may even be toxic to the liver. Check out the list of herbs in Table 13.1, then, if you decide to take herbal supplements, play it safe, and talk to your doctor.

TABLE 13.1: COMMON HERBAL TREATMENTS

Name of Herb	Common Uses
Alfalfa	Used to boost the immune system, help build strong muscles, and gain weight.
Aloe Vera	Taken internally to relieve constipation, gastritis, and stomach ulcers.
Angelica (Dong Quai)	Boosts production of red blood cells and treats weakness and fatigue. Stimulates immune system.
Astragalus	Stimulates the immune system and boosts white blood cell activity. Increases the production of interferon.
Bee Pollen	Balances the endocrine system, helps to relieve prostate problems. Helps to counteract the effects of aging and strengthens the body's natural immunity against illness.
Borage	Stimulates adrenal glands and helps to restore energy.
Burdock Root	Promotes healthy kidney function and helps to prevent water retention.
Capsicum	Helps to increase thermogenesis for weight loss, especially when combined with caffeine-type herbs, and increases heart action without increasing blood pressure.
Cat's Claw	Contains powerful antioxidants that fight free radicals, which set the stage for cancer. Keeps blood platelets from clumping together and helps to prevent strokes and heart attack.
Chamomile	Depresses the central nervous system and may also aid in boosting immune power. Increases relaxation and promotes quality sleep.
Chaparral	Calms nerves and improves appetite. Acts against free radicals and may be effective in preventing degenerative diseases associated with aging.
Chives	Contains the phytochemical allicin, which has been found to lower blood pressure, prevent certain types of cancer, and reduce cholesterol.

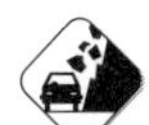

Watch Out! Chaparral has been promoted as a cancer cure and an acne treatment, yet the FDA reports that it has been linked to cases of liver inflammation.

Watch Out!
The FDA recently proposed cracking down on the marketing of Herbal Ecstasy and other ephedra products, citing about 800 illnesses and at least 17 deaths linked to the herbal stimulant. Among the proposals are limiting concentrations of the herb in any dietary supplement, requiring warning labels that its use can cause death, and banning claims that it can help people lose weight or build muscle. Some popular products containing ephedrine include "Herbal Ecstasy," "Ultimate Xphoria," and "Herbal Phen-Fen." It is also marketed as ma huang, Chinese ephedra, and epitonin.

Echinacea	Stimulates the immune system and helps to ward off colds or flu. Heals wounds and has an anti-inflammatory, antiviral, and antibacterial effect in the body.
Evening Primrose	Contains gamma linolenic acid (GLA), an essential nutrient that creates substances called prostaglandins, which help to keep your blood running smoothly. May help to reduce appetite and promote weight loss.
Feverfew	May inhibit inflammation and fever, slows the blood vessel reaction to vasodilators like prostaglandins, and acts similarly to aspirin.
Garlic	Has antimicrobial and immunostimulating properties. Releases a powerful antibiotic called allicin. May lower blood pressure and prevent blood clots.
Ginger	Stimulates mucus-producing vagus nerve reflexes. Has nearly a dozen antiviral compounds, an antioxidant effect, and an anti-inflammatory effect. Stimulates the production of interferon.
Ginkgo biloba	Relaxes and opens up blood vessels. May increase male sexual performance and counteract male impotence. Protects cell membranes from free radical damage, improving concentration and memory, increasing blood flow, helping the symptoms of PMS, and helping with depression.
Ginseng	Use to increase energy and relieve stress. May stimulate special enzymes that promote elimination of toxic foreign substances, as well as increase the immune response by stimulating the number of antibodies in the body. Use to stimulate memory, counteract fatigue, and soothe damage caused by stress.
Goldenseal	Soothes inflammation of the respiratory, digestive, and genitourinary tracts caused by allergy or infection.
Goto kola	Use as "brain food" to improve memory, alleviate mental fatigue, and normalize blood pressure. Considered to be a nerve tonic.

Hawthorn Berries	Use to strengthen the muscles and nerves to the heart. May help regulate high or low blood pressure and battle arteriol-sclerosis, hypoglycemia, and heart disease.
Hyssop	Regulates blood pressure and promotes circulation. Use to relieve hoarseness, lung congestion, and mucus buildup.
Kava Kava	Used to fend off anxiety and nervous tension. Effective as a sedative, diuretic, and muscle relaxant. As an anti-inflammatory, it is used as a pain reliever to replace aspirin, acetaminophen, or ibuprofen.
Kelp	Provides energy and endurance, helps to relieve nervous tension, and promotes circulation to the brain.
Lavender	Relieves insomnia, depression, and headache.
Licorice	Use as an antiulcer drug, antibacterial, and decay-preventive. Promotes healthy adrenal glands and acts as a sexual stimulant. Induces the adrenal cortex to produce more cortisone.
Meadowsweet	Use to ease the pain of arthritis or rheumatism.
Milk Thistle	Increases levels of glutathione, the main vehicle of detoxification in the body. Bolsters the immune system.
Myrrh	Cleans the colon and soothes digestive system upset.
Nettle	Use to relieve arthritis, gout, eczema, hemorrhoids, hay fever, and diarrhea. Has a diuretic effect.
Passionflower	Used frequently as a mild tranquilizer and to ease insomnia, stress, and anxiety. Relieves shingles, hiccups, and asthma.
Peppermint	Aids in digestion, soothes the lining of the digestive tract, and stimulates the production of bile.
Psyllium	Helps to restore tone to the intestines and also lubricates and heals irritated tissues. Used as a natural laxative and cleans out the colon of accumulated toxic debris.

Bright Idea
A recent study of the effects of ginkgo biloba on impotence shows that it boosts blood flow to the penis and brain; after nine months of treatment with ginkgo, 78 percent of impotent men regained their erections, including all those who had previously been helped by impotence drugs.

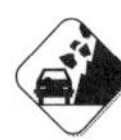

Watch Out! Herbal supplements may not be what the labels claim and active ingredients may vary. According to Consumer Reports, a test of 10 brands of ginseng showed the concentration of ginsenoside—the active ingredient—varied from brand to brand, with some pills having 20 times as much as others.

Pycnogenol	Antioxidant that is said to boost the action of serotonin in the body. Contains a special blend of water-soluble bioflavonoids to boost immune function and reduce the formation of histamine and inflammation.
Saw Palmetto	Used as a treatment for benign prostatic hypertrophy or enlarged prostate by relieving the main symptom of frequent urination.
Slippery Elm	Relieves sore throats and soothes mucous membranes. Helps heal ulcers and relieves heartburn and common digestive complaints.
Spirulina	Aids in weight control, allergies, and anemia. Boosts the immune system, reduces cholesterol, and aids mineral absorption.
St. John's Wort	Used internally to relieve depression without the serious side effects of prescription antidepressants. Used externally to aid in wound healing.
Turmeric	Stimulates the flow of bile and helps to digest fats. Aids digestion, treats dysentery, wards off ulcers, and protects the liver. May combat certain cancers. Helps to prevent heart disease by lowering cholesterol and may prevent the formation of blood clots that trigger heart attacks and strokes.
Valerian	Used to relieve stress and nervousness. Has a sedative effect and has been shown to help in treating insomnia.

Homeopathy may help

Homeopathy is a naturopathic form of medicine that is based on the principle of "like cures, like symptoms," which means that remedies that would cause a potential problem in large doses will actually encourage the body to heal more rapidly if given in small doses. Homeopathetic remedies are made from plant, animal, or mineral substances, and are regulated by the Food and Drug Administration (FDA).

Homeopathic medicines may be helpful in treating allergies, hay fever, migraine headaches, trauma, gastritis, allergic asthma, acute childhood diarrhea, fibromyalgia, and influenza. Some common homeopathic remedies are given in Table 13.2.

TABLE 13.2: COMMON HOMEOPATHIC REMEDIES

Remedy	Ailments
Arnica	Sore muscles, bruises, sprains
Chamomilla	Irritability, depression, anxiety
Cimicifuga	Anxiety, depression
Cocculus	Depression, sleep deprivation
Colocynthis	Irritability, anger, depression
Dioscorea villosa	Irritability
Ignatia amara	Depression, sadness
Ipecacuanha	Irritability, moodiness
Nux vomica	Diarrhea, hemorrhoids, anxiety, oversensitivity.
Sepia	Depression, moodiness

Deletions as per author.

- The Upside: While homeopathy may not correct your impotence, a survey of 107 clinical trials published in the *British Medical Journal* (February, 1991) showed that 80 percent were in favor of homeopathy. Other studies in British journals provided evidence that homeopathic remedies are beneficial in treating allergies, asthma, migraine, flu, and hay fever. One landmark review published in *The Lancet* said that homeopathy was shown to be nearly 2 $^1/_2$ times more effective than placebos in the treatment of such problems as arthritis, allergies, varicose veins, and gastrointestinal pain. In this case, homeopathic remedies may replace medications that have impotence as a side effect for such problems as chronic pain or allergies.

Watch Out!
The Massachusetts Male Aging Study (MMAS) looked at 1,700 Boston-area men, ages 40 to 70, and found that impotence in middle-aged and older men was almost always linked to vascular conditions such as heart disease, hypertension, and diabetes. Smoking and alcoholism also affected impotence but, interestingly enough, not testosterone.

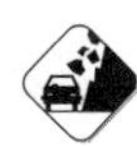

Watch Out!
The FDA lists nine herbs that are considered unsafe: chaparral, comfrey, germander, jin bu huan, lobelia, magnolia, ma huang, stephania, and yohimbine.

- The Downside: Lack of convincing scientific proof is one of the great problems with homeopathy's acceptance by conventional medical doctors. Critics believe that because the medications are so diluted, the only benefit received is placebo.

You will need an initial consultation with a homeopathic practitioner; then check in with this person as needed. Dosing is individualized, depending on what ailment you are trying to relieve. It usually takes two to three days of treatment to notice any change in condition. If you do not find relief within this period, try another remedy. Because some homeopathic remedies are derived from plants, they can be toxic if taken whole.

The bottom line on homeopathy is that although it is increasing in popularity, this type of alternative medical treatment has always received great scrutiny by the traditional medical community. If you seek advice from a homeopathic practitioner, be sure this person is a medical doctor. Ask where he or she has studied homeopathy and whether a certification exam was passed. Licensing is only required in three states at this time, and there are no formal guidelines or formal schools for homeopathy. Because of the possibility of allergic reactions, it is also imperative that you check with your own physician before taking any unknown substance or supplement that promises great cures.

Seek Medical Help First

If you are thinking about trying alternative therapies for ending impotence, it's a good idea to first get a good workup with your family doctor or a board certified urologist. Also consider talking with a qualified psychologist, marriage and family counselor, or social worker to fully evaluate the causes of impotence.

Always ask questions about any alternative treatment before you take it. You might consider the following:

- How old is the treatment? (If it is new, find out the facts before you use it. There are many health sites on the Internet that give detailed factual information about herbs and other alternative therapies.)
- Is it approved by the Food and Drug Administration? (The FDA requires extensive testing for drugs but herbs, for the most part, are tested only for toxicity. Plus, herbal treatments are not regulated. But it does give some reassurance if the treatment has been formally approved after scientific trials.)
- What are the ingredients? (Make a list of the contents and dosages, and ask your pharmacist about the treatment's safety.)
- What are the side effects? (Just like prescription medications, some non-standard treatments have dangerous side effects; others do not.)
- What are the chances for improvement? (If the practitioner claims that this is a "miracle" cure, it is best to walk away. Real miraculous breakthroughs are very few, and a responsible scientist would not call such a breakthrough a "miracle.")
- How much does it cost? (Some alternative treatments may not be reimbursable by your health insurance provider.)
- Can it be taken with traditional medical treatment? (Avoid treatments that require you to stop any medication your conventional doctor has prescribed for you.)

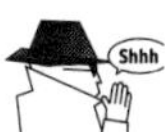

Unofficially... Homeopathic sales are rapidly growing, by 25 percent a year, according to the National Center for Homeopathy.

While you can experience positive results with alternative therapies, there may also be some side effects such as low blood pressure, increased anxiety, abdominal distress, elevated heart rate, or kidney disease, depending on treatments you might take. This does not mean that you will have these side effects; but in order to be safe, check with your doctor about any alternative treatment.

The outlook for alternative treatments is remarkably optimistic, and some of these may help you regain connections among your mind, body, and spirit, as well as increase good health, prevent disease, and eliminate impotence. Yet keep in mind that the safest way to stay well is to rely upon your conventional medical doctor. Then invest in your total health with a wellness program that blends the conventional modes of therapy with safe, alternative treatments. After all, why not take advantage of the best of both worlds?

Just the Facts

- Alternative medicine focuses on mind/body interplay and the link among outside stressors, our emotions, and physical health.

- Because impotence can be related to a stressful lifestyle, it may be easily treated with alternative therapies.

- Some herbs such as St. John's Wort may help ease depression, while saw palmetto can help reduce an enlarged prostate.

Chapter 14

GET THE SCOOP ON...

Certain foods that are supposed to be sexual stimulants ■ Why obesity can add to erectile dysfunction ■ How the Body Mass Index (BMI) relates to your risk of serious illness ■ The relationship between libido and foods high in zinc

Overcoming Impotence Naturally

Throughout history, man has searched for natural ways to boost sexual pleasures. You've probably read stories of people eating foods that remind them of genitalia, from phallic-looking roots and animal horns, to soft and moist peaches, oysters, or tomatoes, hoping they were sexual stimulants. Other reports pertain to certain vitamins or even exercise that research has found to make sex more satisfying.

While the jury is still out on any magical cure for impotence, there are a host of lifestyle changes you can make to increase healthy erectile function—and decrease the chances of health problems such as heart disease, diabetes, and hypertension, all of which can lead to impotence.

Changing Bad Habits

As you have read, impotence can be linked to obesity that is caused by overeating and lack of exercise, cigarette smoking, and alcohol use, among other

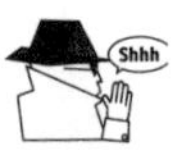

Unofficially... Researchers suggest that several dietary aphrodisiacs, including yohimbine, oysters, rosemary, ginseng, caffeine, ginkgo biloba, and chocolate, do stimulate more than just the imagination.

lifestyle habits. The good news is that getting in control of all these habits (or risk factors) is possible—and it is not that hard.

Impotence and obesity

Obesity is defined as being 20 percent or more over normal body weight and affects one-third of the U.S. population. According to a Louis Harris and Associates survey in 1997, Americans are fatter than ever before. Seventy-four percent of Americans 25 or older are overweight, up from 71 percent in 1996, 69 percent in 1994, 66 percent in 1992, and 59 percent 10 years ago. That extra poundage can mean increased risk of heart disease, high blood pressure, diabetes, stroke, gallbladder disease, arthritis, sleep and breathing problems, and some types of cancer.

Not only does being overweight make it difficult to be an agile lover (and much less sexy to look at!), weighing as little as 10 or 15 pounds over your recommended weight can exacerbate a heart condition, elevate blood pressure and cholesterol, and even increase your risk of certain cancers. Obesity is a major risk factor for obstructive sleep apnea (OSA), which increases the chance of impotence, and it makes it more difficult to breathe.

By now you know that serious ailments such as hypertension and heart disease and the medications used to treat these may lead to erectile dysfunction. Yet many people find that their disease can be controlled by less medication when they lose excess pounds.

In the midst of the pessimistic outlook for overweight men, there is some good news. While being obese can increase the chance of impotence, as well as serious illness, losing weight can reduce your risk.

Check your BMI

Newer research on obesity indicates that your body mass index (BMI) gives a more accurate picture of health than simply using scales. The BMI number correlates to your risk of adverse effects on health, with higher numbers showing an increased risk. According to the American Dietetic Association, people with a higher percentage of body fat tend to have a higher BMI than those who have a greater percentage of muscle. It is this extra body fat, not muscle, that puts you at greater risk for health problems.

Using the BMI chart (see Figure 14.1), locate the weight closest to your weight in the left-hand column. Then locate the height closest to your height along the top. Where these two numbers meet on the chart is your BMI. For example, if you weigh 180 pounds and are 5' 8" tall, your BMI according to this chart is 27. Keep in mind that each man is different. Your weight can depend on many variables, including your height, age, and bone structure. The best weight for you is the one where you are healthy and, hopefully, do not have impotence!

> "Forget the scales. It only takes a quick glance in the mirror to know when I've gained some weight.
> —Paul, teacher, 42"

TABLE 14.1: BMI INDEX

BMI	Risk for Health Problems Related to Body Weight
20–25	Very low risk
26–30	Low risk
31–35	Moderate risk
36-40	High risk
40+	Very high risk

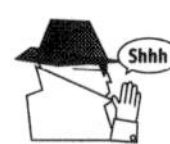

Unofficially... The BMI is defined as body weight (in kilograms) divided by height (in square meters).

FIGURE 14.1: BODY MASS INDEX (BMI)

Body Mass Index (BMI)
Height (ft, in)

Weight (lb)	4'10"	4'11"	5'0"	5'1"	5'2"	5'3"	5'4"	5'5"	5'6"	5'7"	5'8"	5'9"	5'10"	5'11"	6'0"	6'1"	6'2"
125	26	25	24	24	23	22	22	21	20	20	19	18	18	17	17	17	16
130	27	26	25	25	24	23	22	22	21	20	20	19	19	18	18	17	17
135	28	27	26	26	25	24	23	23	22	21	21	20	19	19	18	18	17
140	29	28	27	27	26	25	24	23	23	22	21	21	20	20	19	19	18
145	30	29	28	27	27	26	25	24	23	23	22	21	21	20	20	19	19
150	31	30	29	28	27	27	26	25	24	24	23	22	22	21	20	20	19
155	32	31	30	29	28	28	27	26	25	24	24	23	22	22	21	20	20
160	34	32	31	30	29	28	28	27	26	25	24	24	23	22	22	21	21
165	35	33	32	31	30	29	28	28	27	26	25	24	24	23	22	22	21
170	36	34	33	32	31	30	29	28	28	27	26	25	24	24	23	22	22
175	37	35	34	33	32	31	30	29	28	27	27	26	25	24	24	23	23
180	38	36	35	34	33	32	31	30	29	28	27	27	26	25	25	24	23
185	39	37	36	35	34	33	32	31	30	29	28	27	27	26	25	24	24
190	40	38	37	36	35	34	33	32	31	30	29	28	27	27	26	25	24
195	41	39	38	37	36	35	34	33	32	31	30	29	28	27	27	26	25
200	42	40	39	38	37	36	34	33	32	31	30	30	29	28	27	26	26
205	43	41	40	39	38	36	35	34	33	32	31	30	29	29	28	27	26
210	44	43	41	40	38	37	36	35	34	33	32	31	30	29	29	28	27
215	45	44	42	41	39	38	37	36	35	34	33	32	31	30	29	28	28
220	46	45	43	42	40	39	38	37	36	35	34	33	32	31	30	29	28
225	47	46	44	43	41	40	39	38	36	35	34	33	32	31	31	30	29
230	48	47	45	44	42	41	40	38	37	36	35	34	33	32	31	30	30
235	49	48	46	44	43	42	40	39	38	37	36	35	34	33	32	31	30
240	50	49	47	45	44	43	41	40	39	38	37	36	35	34	33	32	31
245	51	50	48	46	45	43	42	41	40	38	37	36	35	34	33	32	32
250	52	51	49	47	46	44	43	42	40	39	38	37	36	35	34	33	32
255	53	52	50	48	47	45	44	43	41	40	39	38	37	36	35	34	33
260	54	53	51	49	48	46	45	43	42	41	40	38	37	36	35	34	33
265	56	54	52	50	49	47	46	44	43	42	40	39	38	37	36	35	34
270	57	55	53	51	49	48	46	45	44	42	41	40	39	38	37	36	35
275	58	56	54	52	50	49	47	46	44	43	42	41	40	38	37	36	35
280	59	57	55	53	51	50	48	47	45	44	43	41	40	39	38	37	36
285	60	58	56	54	52	51	49	48	46	45	43	42	41	40	39	38	37
290	61	59	57	55	53	51	50	48	47	46	44	43	42	41	39	38	37
295	62	60	58	56	54	52	51	49	48	46	45	44	42	41	40	39	38
300	63	61	59	57	55	53	52	50	48	47	46	44	43	42	41	40	39
305	64	62	60	58	56	54	52	51	49	48	46	45	44	43	41	40	39
310	65	63	61	59	57	55	53	52	50	49	47	46	45	43	42	41	40
315	66	64	62	60	58	56	54	53	51	49	48	47	45	44	43	42	41
320	67	65	63	61	59	57	55	53	52	50	49	47	46	45	43	42	41
325	68	66	64	62	60	58	56	54	53	51	50	48	47	45	44	43	42

Move around more

The best way to maintain or reach an ideal weight is to burn more calories than you take in via exercise and activity. Researchers have found that among those who are successful at keeping off the weight, more than 95 percent are exercisers—and most are walkers. So, besides using the BMI to figure out if you are at risk for serious illness, you also need to calculate how many calories you need to burn to lose extra pounds. Check out Table 14.2 to see how many calories are burned by various activities.

TABLE 14.2: COMMON WAYS TO BURN 200 CALORIES A DAY*

Activity	Minutes to Burn 200 Calories	Activity	Minutes to Burn 200 Calories
Aerobics (high/ low impact)	20	Bicycling (12 mph)	22
Cleaning	54	Cooking	72
Dancing (slow)	68	Jogging (5 mph)	26
Making beds	82	Mowing lawn (power)	58
Stationary cycling (10 mph)	32	Tennis (doubles)	52
Vacuuming	34	Walking (3 mph)	54
Walking (4 mph)	36	Watching television	154
Weight training	40	Weeding garden	38

*Based on a 130-pound person

If the thought of working out makes you run—the other way—you are not alone.

Nonetheless, moving around more with exercise will help you lose weight and that will decrease your risk of serious diseases, as well as help you be a more fit and appealing partner. Check out the benefits of exercise listed below:

- Increases metabolism to burn more calories
- Improves the quality of sleep
- Reduces body fat

Bright Idea
Studies show that men burn about 60 calories for every 10 minutes of passionate sex. Maybe this is more incentive to lose weight, add exercise, and end impotence!

Watch Out!
Be careful riding that old 10-speed! New studies show that sitting on an ordinary narrow, pointed seat can crush an artery (the cavernosal artery) that controls the ability of the penis to fill with blood. Research confirms that impotence happens more often to cyclists than to runners. To avoid the problem, make sure the seat is level—not tilted up or down—and rise up before you hit a bump in the road.

- Fights aging
- Boosts brain power
- Helps to protect against cancer
- Strengthens your bones
- Boosts endorphins, improving mood and helping to relieve depression
- Cuts your risk for diabetes, hypertension, and other diseases
- Improves cholesterol profile (increases protective HDLs)
- Enhances your self-image
- Increases your sexual appetite (libido)

Stopping cigarettes

Cigarette smoking is a major risk factor for coronary heart disease, especially heart attack and heart failure. This disease, along with the necessary medications for treatment, places you at higher risk for impotence. Other medical problems related to cigarette smoking include:

- Cancer
- Diabetes
- Osteoporosis
- Atherosclerosis and blockage of the arteries that supply the legs, which can lead to gangrene and amputation
- Atherosclerosis and blockage of the arteries that supply the brain, which can lead to stroke
- Increased risk of sudden death
- Peptic ulcers; smoking may also interfere with the treatment of ulcer disease
- Cancer of the mouth, throat (larynx), esophagus, lungs, kidneys, bladder, and pancreas

- Increased LDL-cholesterol and possibly decreased HDL-cholesterol
- Emphysema and chronic bronchitis (chronic lung disease)
- Coughs, respiratory infections, and asthma illnesses
- Decreased physical performance, endurance, and lung function
- Interference with actions of medications given for other medical problems

Stopping cigarettes may be the most important step you take as you break lifestyle habits that increase your chance of impotence. More on the dangers of smoking will appear later in this chapter.

Bright Idea
Men who have a regular exercise program have a lower risk of developing coronary heart disease than men who are inactive. Exercise is helpful for weight control and relaxation and may raise HDL-cholesterol, the good cholesterol.

Alcohol and erectile dysfunction

Drinking alcohol suppresses the connection from the brain to the penis when you are erotically aroused. Alcohol also increases your risk of serious illness such as diabetes, osteoporosis, heart disease, and liver disease, among others. Knowing this fact, it's important that you drink less—or not at all—if you are having erectile dysfunction after drinking alcohol.

High-Performance Eating

According to the National Institutes of Health (NIH), true weight-loss success can only come from changing eating habits for good—for a lifetime. You already have certain habits, like brushing your teeth, that you do without thinking twice. Eating a low-fat, healthy diet must also become a natural part of your daily life—a true eating habit change that will result in weight loss.

The Food Guide Pyramid (see Figure 14.2) from the United States Dietetic Association provides us with an illustration of how we should eat to stay lean and healthy. It recommends plenty of low-fat, nutrient-dense foods such as fruits, vegetables, cereal, bread, and pasta, with less of an emphasis on whole milk products and high-fat meats. The foundation of our diet, like the pyramid, should be built on the plant foods—fruits, vegetables, and grain products. That does not mean we eliminate the milk and meat or meat substitute groups. You can use low-fat versions of these foods to complement the rest of the plant-based diet. Fats and sweets should be used sparingly, especially in people trying to lose weight, as these contribute extra calories but few nutrients.

"I refuse to ever diet again. I firmly believe that the first three letters in 'diet' is exactly what will happen to me from the deprivation.
—Cameron, doctoral student, 31"

FIGURE 14.2: THE FOOD GUIDE PYRAMID

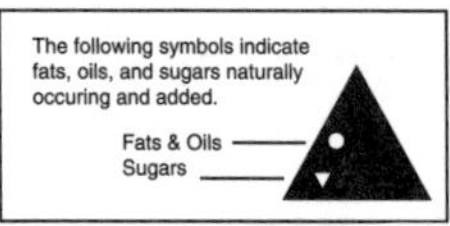

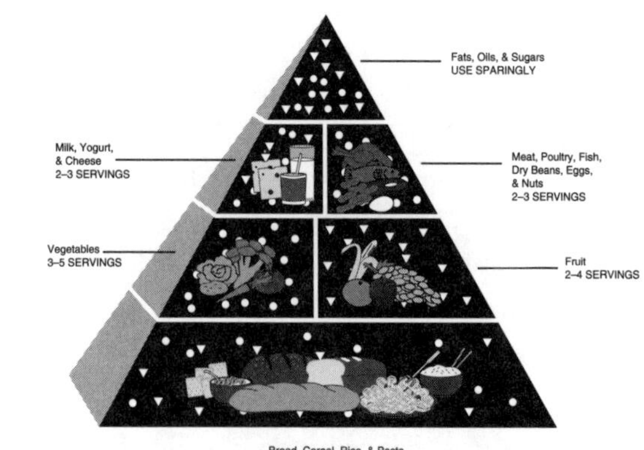

Be sure to follow these guidelines when choosing from the Food Guide Pyramid:

- Choose more servings from the plant groups (bread, cereal, rice, pasta, fruits, and vegetables)
- Choose fewer servings from animal groups (dairy and meat)
- Choose fats and sweets sparingly, especially for weight reduction

Stop dieting and start eating right

If any single diet program or eating style worked for everyone, we would all be thin. As you may have noticed, we're not. So, what may help you get down to a normal weight might not work for your friend or colleague. Because we are all different, some people like to have a specific food plan to follow as they initiate healthy lifestyle changes, while others would rather have the freedom to select foods that appeal to them.

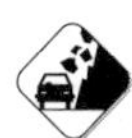

Watch Out!
Some very-low-calorie diets, high-protein diets, and liquid diets are useful in clinical settings, but you need professional supervision and monitoring to use these safely. There are some popular eating "plans" that are actually very healthy and can help you lose weight. If you wish to use one of the described plans, check with your doctor or a certified nutritionist to make sure all your nutritional needs are met.

Remember that calories count

Even though selecting low-fat food choices is the key to weight reduction, not surprisingly, calories still count. The American Dietetic Association recommends a calorie level of no less than ten times your desired weight, with men getting at least 1,400 calories per day. This is good news for those dieters who have tried to maintain very-low-calorie diets with little success. For example, if your goal is 180 pounds, you should eat around 1,800 calories per day. If your goal is 160 pounds, then you can follow a diet of 1,600 calories per day for weight reduction. This daily calorie allowance will not make for a quick weight reduction, but studies show that it is better to make lifestyle changes and lose weight slowly in order to keep it off for good.

Use the following chart to plan your daily weight reduction program; make selections according to the various categories. Table 14.3 uses a desired calorie count of 1,500 as an example. If you need to change this calorie allotment for weight reduction, talk with a certified nutritionist for additional information.

TABLE 14.3: DAILY CALORIE LEVEL OF 1,500 FOR WEIGHT LOSS

Food Groups	Recommended # of Servings
Bread servings	Eight
Fruit servings	Three
Meat servings	Three (six ounces)
Dairy servings	Three (low-fat)
Vegetable servings	Four

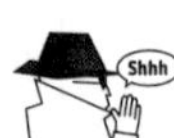

Unofficially... Fat has twice the caloric value of carbohydrates (nine calories per gram of weight versus four calories per gram of weight). Lowering your fat intake will help you notice a significant reduction in calories.

A low-fat diet

A diet low in fat, particularly saturated fat, found in animal products and trans fats, found in pastries and baked goods, can help you reduce your weight as well as your risk of some serious diseases.

While the 10-percent low-fat diet was formulated to heal ailing hearts, it has also been found helpful for cancer prevention and weight loss. Before you start piling on the fruits and vegetables, you must know that the only way you can cut fat to 10 percent of calories is to eliminate more sources of animal protein from your diet.

Probably the safest goal to aim for is 20 to 25 percent total fat calories in your daily diet. While this is still a low-fat diet, there is enough fat to help you feel full after eating. And common sense tells you that if you do not feel full, you are only going to raid the refrigerator later during the football game on TV.

It might help to use the following formula to calculate your goal in grams of fat on a 10-percent, 20-percent, or 30-percent diet, using this method:

- For a 30-percent fat diet, divide your ideal body weight (in pounds) by two.
- For a 20-percent fat diet, divide your ideal body weight by three.
- For a 10-percent fat diet, divide your ideal body weight by six.

For example, if your ideal body weight is 180 pounds, the 30-percent goal allows 90 grams of fat per day, or 180 divided by two; the 20-percent limit is 60 grams; the 10-percent limit is 30 grams.

- Red meat
- Cheese
- Whole milk
- Butter
- Hydrogenated fats

Timesaver
If you have no time to prepare fresh vegetables, take advantage of the pre-packaged produce at the grocery store. Broccoli, cauliflower, spinach, and many types of salad mixes are available in single servings or larger.

A diet high in fruits and vegetables

A diet high in fiber, consisting of fruits, vegetables, lentils, nuts, and seeds, will keep you full and also help you get rid of extra weight.

Only a fistful

No matter how you decide to change your poor eating habits, portion control is still important. You may eat nothing but fruits and vegetables, but if you eat more calories than you burn off, you will not budge on the scales. In fact, you may notice a weight gain!

Check out the Food Guide Pyramid serving sizes, then compare these with what you are now eating. If you are unsure as to what comprises two to three ounces of meat, it is about as much as fits in the palm of your hand.

Keep score

No matter how you change your eating habits, it may help you to write down everything you eat in a "food journal." Keeping a journal will help you know exactly where you stand nutritionally. You may think you are eating a healthful diet, watching your portions; then after calculating your calories at the end of the day, you find that you have eaten twice as many as you thought.

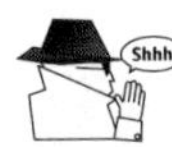

Unofficially... Fourteen million Americans claim to be strict vegetarians, while more than 46 percent or 120 million Americans are reducing meat consumption.

TABLE 14.4: FOOD GUIDE PYRAMID SERVING SIZES

Bread, Cereal, Rice, and Pasta
One slice of bread
1/2 hamburger bun
1/2 bagel
1/2 English muffin
3/4 ounce of pretzels
1/2 cup cooked cereal, pasta, or rice
One ounce cold cereal

Milk
One cup skim or non-fat milk
One cup non-fat, sugar-free yogurt
1-1/2 ounce fat-free cheese

Meat and Meat Substitutes
Two to three ounces of lean meat, fish, or poultry without the skin
One cup to 1-1/2 cup cooked beans
Two eggs or 1/2 cup low-cholesterol egg alternative

Fruit
One medium piece of fruit
1/2 cup chopped, cooked, or canned fruit
1/2 cup fruit juice

Vegetables
1/2 cup cooked
One cup raw

Some helpful hints

It's not painful to control the foods you eat. In fact, sometimes all you need to do is make adjustments such as changing from whole milk to low-fat milk or using no-fat mayonnaise in your tuna salad instead of regular mayonnaise. No matter what your weight is, it is also helpful to discuss any dietary changes with a certified nutritionist. Ask your doctor for a referral. Some easy-to-implement nutritional tips to lower fat and calories are given in Chapter 5.

Think zinc

Researchers believe that the more sexually active a man is, the more zinc he will need. It appears that zinc helps to regulate testosterone levels, which dictate a man's sexual appetite. Also, if you exercise regularly and intensely, you may also need more zinc. For example, in studies, runners have lower plasma zinc levels than control subjects.

While a substantial amount of zinc is lost in perspiration, increasing the calcium intake in the body can inhibit zinc absorption. Foods high in iron also compete with zinc.

Zinc also has antioxidant effects and is vital to the body's resistance to infection and for tissue repair. Many illnesses, such as some cancers, kidney disease, long-term infection, trauma, and cirrhosis of the liver, are associated with zinc deficiency. Medications may also interfere with absorption in the intestines and cause a zinc deficiency.

The Recommended Dietary Allowance (RDA) for zinc is 15 mg for men. Foods high in zinc include seafood, eggs, meats, whole grains, wheat germ, nuts, and seeds; tea and coffee may hinder absorption. Check with your physician for what is safe in your situation.

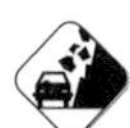

Watch Out! Excessive amounts of zinc are toxic. Too much interferes with metabolism of other minerals in the body, particularly iron and copper.

Starting the Exercise Habit

Exercise does more than just keep your muscles strong and your heart ticking. Studies show that moving around more with exercise actually restores the body's neurochemical balance, which affects our emotional state. In studies, women reported a dramatic increase in sexual activity and arousal after beginning a regular exercise program. Not only were they more physically fit, but their stress levels were also greatly reduced, helping to enhance their sex lives. Of course, we feel certain that these studies would be just as positive for men! In this regard, perhaps exercise is the "aerobic aphrodisiac." Now that's incentive to begin moving around more!

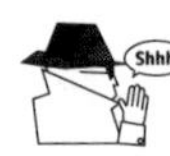

Unofficially... According to the Centers for Disease Control and Prevention (CDC), 56 percent of men and 44 percent of women between ages 18 and 29 exercise regularly. These numbers drop to 44 percent and 40 percent, respectively, among people 30 to 44.

Research has also shown that regular participation in aerobic training has been reported to reduce symptoms of moderate depression and enhance psychological fitness.

What else can exercise do?

- Produce changes in the chemical levels in the body, which can have an affect on your psychological state.
- Raise plasma levels of endorphins and may help to alleviate symptoms of depression.
- Slow down heart-racing epinephrine (adrenaline)
- Help you maintain a normal weight
- Increase longevity
- Decrease your chance of chronic illness.

The exercise/stress connection

Exercise increases alpha waves that are associated with relaxation and meditation; exercise also acts as a displacement defense mechanism. How does this work? You may get up early each day to deal with your career and children, then after working hard all day, not get into bed until late at night. This ongoing daily stress and lack of healthful sleep might cause you to become more irritable and quick tempered around your partner.

But exercise can help. Most studies now show that exercise can help direct the anxiety and emotions away and help you gain some hopeful feelings about yourself and your relationship. If you have ever participated in a lengthy period of aerobics or walked for several miles, perhaps you know the benefit of this displacement defense mechanism. Isn't it difficult to worry about daily stresses or even relationship battles when you are working hard physically? All that is on your mind is getting through the routine—and not the problems you face each day. No matter what your age or how busy you are, you can incorporate a regular exercise routine into your daily life.

Making a commitment

While you may agree that exercise is beneficial, many people feel that conditioning is for the young. However, studies show that everyone—even senior citizens—can benefit greatly from movement and exercise. One study tested a group of 100 frail nursing home patients over a period of time. Those who received exercise training increased muscle strength and gait velocity; their ability to climb stairs improved. Those patients who did not receive exercise training remained the same or declined in strength. This study concluded that even the frail elderly greatly benefit from exercise as a means to counteract muscle weakness and physical frailty. If the frail elderly can show physical improvement from exercise, imagine what exercise will do for you!

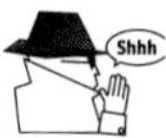

Unofficially... Government statistics show that 60 percent of all Americans get no regular exercise, a statistic that has remained steady for the last two decades. While exercise can cost nothing and is the key to maintaining a normal weight, isn't it ironic that $30 billion is spent on diet foods and diet programs each year by the American public?

A daily habit

Finding the time to exercise may seem more difficult than actually performing the activity, but once you begin an exercise program, and while it takes time to reach this level, you will be surprised how you will depend on it. You will find your overall performance improves in every area of your life—career, relationships with other people, and relationships at home. You may even get another boost—performance in the bedroom may improve! Some men even tell of adding another day of exercise on their "day off" because they enjoy the boost of endorphins, the body's natural pain relievers, that aerobic training gives them. Rest is also important to a regular exercise program, so be sure to get enough.

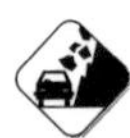

Watch Out!
A word of caution: If you have not been physically active, be sure to consult your physician before starting any exercise program.

It may take you weeks to months to get a routine established. While an ongoing, daily exercise program will help you to see some short-term results of improved moods, it may take longer to really see the benefit of weight control and greater energy.

Take baby steps

Go slowly at first, and then pick up your pace as you are able. Starting small, then building into a full exercise program will help you become adjusted to the exercise and help you to make it a habit. For example, if you are healthy, and start out walking and swimming as your exercise, start with just 10 minutes a day the first week. As you increase in strength and endurance, add five minutes the second week, then another five minutes the third week, and on until you get up to an acceptable program.

Do what you enjoy

Be sure to choose those activities that you enjoy and do them in moderation—both in time spent and in intensity. One reason people drop exercise programs is that they get bored; either the exercise becomes too mundane, the scenery is too repetitious, or the results are not startling enough to keep them motivated. Another reason people quit exercising is that they try to do too much too soon and instead of receiving aerobic benefits, they become injured.

Stopping Cigarettes

Perhaps of all the bad habits you have—from overeating to being a couch potato—smoking cigarettes is the most dangerous. In simplest terms—cigarette smoking will kill you.

Why you have to quit

Each year, more than 390,000 people die from the effects of cigarette smoking. More than 3,000 of these deaths are from lung cancer directly attributable to tobacco smoke.

Smoking greatly raises the risk of all types of health problems, including diabetes, osteoporosis, some types of cancer, hypertension, heart disease, emphysema, and chronic bronchitis, among others. According to the American Lung Association, current male smokers over age 35 are 10 times more likely to die of chronic obstructive pulmonary disease (COPD) and 22 more times more likely to die of lung cancer than non-smoking males.

Enough statistics. If you smoke, you know how it can harm you. No one needs to tell you of the increased risk of serious or even terminal illness. But cigarette smoking also hinders erections—and stopping cigarettes may allow you to perform sexually the way you would like.

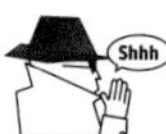

Unofficially... While in the United States, 1.5 million quit smoking each year, as many as 50 million adults continue to smoke. Perhaps an even more disturbing statistic is that each day in the United States, more than 2,000 teenagers start to smoke for the first time. In fact, some revealing studies state that more than one-third of all high school students currently smoke cigarettes.

Plan to quit

While it usually takes a serious disease to make someone quit smoking, you can get a head start at improving, and maybe even saving, your life, if you make a commitment today to stop. It must be recognized that cigarettes contain nicotine, a stimulant and addicting drug. After you stop cigarettes, you may experience irritability, nervousness, and headaches for one to two weeks, especially if you have been a heavy smoker. The newer non-prescription nicotine patches that are worn on the skin, nicotine gum, or other medications can help you through the difficult period of withdrawal, helping to make the physical problem less troublesome.

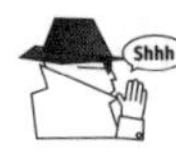

Unofficially... While most studies state that 45 consecutive minutes of conditioning exercise is necessary to get a cardiovascular benefit, there are some new studies that say the daily workout does not have to be done all in the same time. These studies report that you can get the same benefit from 10-minute segments of exercise, three to four times a day, as you do from 45 consecutive minutes.

It is important to remember that even for those who have stopped smoking for years, the urge to smoke can always return. It is a matter of mental self-control to avoid cigarettes. Having the emotional support of a spouse, family, and understanding friends and coworkers is very important.

Soon after quitting, your ability to exercise will increase—even people who have smoked for years may notice an improvement in heart rate, blood pressure, and circulation to the hands, legs, and feet. Think of how much easier it will be to breathe when you are involved intimately with the one you love! If you have trouble stopping smoking, talk to your doctor or call your local chapter of the American Lung Association or the American Cancer Society.

Just the Facts

- Impotence can be linked to habits such as cigarette smoking and alcohol use, and to obesity that is caused by overeating and lack of exercise.
- True weight loss can only come from eating a low-fat, healthy diet that is a natural part of your daily life, eating habits that you do without thinking twice.
- Zinc regulates testosterone levels, which dictate a man's sexual appetite, and is found in eggs, whole grains, and meat.
- Exercise boosts alpha waves that are associated with relaxation and meditation and acts as a displacement defense mechanism.

PART V

The Impotence Solution

Chapter 15

GET THE SCOOP ON...
Your primary care doctor may have answers ▪ Specific risk factors for erectile dysfunction ▪ Options for treatment your doctor can prescribe ▪ Why surgery gives hope to many

Talking with Your Doctor

What do I say?
How do I start the conversation?
Who can I talk with openly?

These are common concerns men have when they discover they are impotent. But there are ample opportunities to get good help and relief for this common condition—if you make the first call.

Start with Your Doctor

Your first contact for information about erectile dysfunction may be during a routine visit to your primary care physician or family doctor. If you are visiting for another problem or having an annual exam, it is a good time to mention that you also would like to talk about treatments for erection problems.

Not a new topic

Keep in mind that this is now a common topic in primary care offices, so try not to feel uncomfortable bringing it up. If you have a routine examination or

> "While most patients go alone on the first visit to discuss erectile dysfunction, if you and your partner feel comfortable, it can sometimes be helpful to go together. Or, you may want to include your partner in the later visits.
> —Jack, urologist, 53"

yearly check-up, your doctor may initiate discussion by asking you about any sexual problems on a written list of questions.

Things get easier once the doctor knows you want specific information. If you let the doctor know it's important to you to get relief, you will definitely see results.

Choosing the best doctor for treatment

If your primary care physician doesn't feel he's the best physician to treat your erectile dysfunction, you may be referred to a urologist. Since urologists specialize in problems of the genital and urinary systems, some men feel better making the first appointment directly with a urologist. If you don't know where to start, call the local medical association and ask for some names of doctors who specialize in erectile dysfunction and impotence.

If your primary care doctor refers you to a urologist or if you decide to start with a urologist, you should feel comfortable from the first phone call. Many offices send booklets or information about their operations and may include a written list of questions you can complete before your visit. This can be an easy way to answer some personal questions about your sex life.

Involve your spouse or partner

This may also be a good opportunity to open communication and to let your partner take part in solving the problem. Very often, a partner actually feels guilty because she is not able to arouse her husband, or she worries that her husband may be involved with a different partner. It is almost always recommended for your partner to have a part in choosing a treatment for the erectile dysfunction. This participation is likely to produce better results in the long run.

Q&A

Your doctor will ask questions to help decide the causes of your erectile dysfunction. For example, be prepared to describe your problem as completely as possible. Be honest, open, and specific—your doctor is used to hearing of these problems many times each day. There will be questions about your general health to learn if any medical problems are causing the erectile dysfunction. Your doctor will also ask about surgery, especially in the back, prostate, or other genital areas. He or she will need to know which medications you're taking.

Of course, there will be questions about your sexual activity, when erections occur, and when difficulty first started. It will be important for your doctor to understand what kind of stress you are under, and this may include problems that you may be having in your relationship with your partner, other possible problems at home, and problems at work. Other risk factors that will be discussed are listed below.

Almost every case of impotence can be successfully treated, but the treatments are different depending on the cause of your erectile dysfunction. The more accurate information you provide to your doctor, the better the treatment he can provide.

For example, you may be asked about your sexual desire, ejaculations, and orgasms. You may be asked questions about your sexual partner. You will be asked about erections during the night, since most men have two or more erections during the night but may not be aware of them. There are some simple ways to tell if you've had erections during sleep.

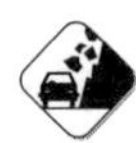

Watch Out!
Keep tabs on your stress because emotional concerns such as fear of failure, problems with your partner, depression, and anger can all increase your chance of erectile dysfunction.

Many of the questions relate to medical problems that increase the risk of erectile dysfunction. As discussed earlier in this book, some of the most common medical problems that contribute to impotence include:

- Diabetes mellitus
- Heavy alcohol use
- Peripheral vascular disease
- Medication side effects
- Damage to nerves that supply the penis (from injuries, diseases, or surgery to the spinal cord, prostate, or pelvis)
- Smoking cigarettes
- Age (over 40–45)
- Hypertension
- Deformities of the penis, such as Peyronie's disease
- Life's stressors

The Physical Examination

Your doctor will perform a physical examination, with an interest in finding any specific problems in the areas involved in sexual function. This means making sure there are no problems with the penis, the prostate, or the testicles. The nerves to the genital area and penis are checked in simple, nonpainful tests. Even though it's important for erection, it is not easy in a physical exam to accurately measure blood supply to the penis. However, the arterial supply to the legs and feet is easily tested and, if abnormal, may indicate limited arterial circulation to the penis.

Your doctor will most likely suggest a number of tests. These could include: a basic blood test to check for other medical problems including diabetes; a test to check testosterone levels, especially if lack of desire, or waning libido, is a symptom; a test to determine the specific blood flow to the penis. This last test may be done by using ultrasound blood flow testing, which can tell the quality of blood flow in the arteries and in the veins of the penis. Another way of testing erection capability is by injection of a medication into the penis to cause an erection, which is limited in those who have certain physical problems, for example, diabetes.

> "Viagra changed my 40-year marriage from dull and boring into a honeymoon again. We're in our late fifties and feel like we are newlyweds.
> —Paul, insurance adjuster, 57"

After these tests, your doctor will probably discuss the possibilities for treatment of your erectile dysfunction. With the many treatments available (as discussed in Chapters 11 through 14), it is possible for almost every patient to find a cure.

After the first visit, your doctor may suggest a trial of Viagra if there are no medical reasons to prevent its use. Viagra is discussed fully in Chapter 11.

Your doctor may suggest injection treatments. If he does recommend this treatment, you will be taught how to inject your penis (very small needles, and a minor discomfort—really) in the doctor's office. You will then try a small test dose, either at the office or at your home. You will then be asked to grade the quality of your erection so the dose of medication used for the injection can be accurately adjusted to give the best results. You will also be instructed in what to do if the erection is painful or lasts more than four hours. When the proper dose is discovered for the best quality erection, you will be told how often you can use the injections (usually two to three times weekly), along with other precautions.

Unofficially... Studies show that erections measured at night in men over 55 happen at a slower rate than in younger men and the circumference of the penis (which tells how large the penis gets) is smaller.

You may also be shown how to use a vacuum device (as discussed in Chapter 12) and may be fitted with a device for home use. Be sure you fully understand how to use the device before you take it home.

Risk Factors

Be aware that many of your own risk factors that may contribute to erectile dysfunction can be managed to help maintain erections with a few simple steps.

Age

For example, a major risk factor is age. Over age 40 to 50, there are normal changes in the penis that can cause a decrease in erection and increase the risk of erectile dysfunction. Researchers have found that the level of testosterone drops and the number of small muscles (which help erection) present in the penis is lower in older men.

Research indicates that the amount of blood flow into the penis decreases with age. In some cases, the veins that carry blood out of the penis may not sufficiently close, causing an earlier loss of erection. This means that you will be able to achieve an adequate erection, but you will not be able to maintain it for more than a few minutes. However, there are ways to manage this problem.

Alcohol and drugs

Drinking alcohol can lower the ability to have an erection. Even though "in the movies" alcohol seems at first to relax, remove inhibitions, and increase sexual function, the truth is that more often as the amount of alcohol consumed increases, the sensitivity of the penis and the reactions of the brain are slowed, which may lower sexual function. Drinking too much before sex may limit performance. One suggestion from sex therapists is to have a drink after sex rather than before, especially if you notice less full erections when you drink.

Drinking large amounts of alcohol over a period of time can also cause erectile dysfunction. It also may have a damaging effect on the testicles and cause problems by lowering the amount and quality of sperm cells. Alcohol also can lower the level of testosterone, which can diminish libido and eventually lessen erections. If you happen to develop liver disease from too much alcohol, then this will likely add to the problems of lower testosterone and erectile dysfunction.

Timesaver
A man past age 40 to 50 may need more direct stimulation to create and maintain an erection.

Use of marijuana, cocaine, or other drugs can affect erections and sexual function. Marijuana can lower testosterone levels and other hormone levels. It also lowers sperm cell numbers. As with other drugs and medications, there may be individual differences in the response.

Diabetes mellitus

Diabetes can cause erection problems when the blood glucose is high. This may be the first sign of diabetes, so it is important to have a medical evaluation if you are experiencing erectile dysfunction. When the blood glucose is brought into normal range, this type of erectile dysfunction goes away.

In men who have had diabetes for years, there can be damage to the nerves that lead to the penis. There may also be less blood supply to the penis, since diabetes increases the risk of atherosclerosis with hardening and narrowing of the arteries. The good news is that complications from these types of problems are often much lower if the blood glucose is controlled properly through diet, exercise, and medication. The goal is to try to keep your blood

Bright Idea
One more of the many benefits of stopping cigarettes may be that your erectile dysfunction improves, along with an increase in life span.

glucose at levels as close as possible to normal, which is possible with the help of your doctor once you know what to do.

Smoking cigarettes

Studies have found that smoking can limit the duration and quality of erections. Animals subjected to cigarette smoke were found to have lower levels of nitric oxide, the chemical critical for erection.

Peripheral vascular disease

Peripheral vascular disease results in blockage of the arteries of the legs, but often also includes blockage of the arteries supplying the penis. The most common cause of this problem is atherosclerosis, which causes hardening and blockage of the arteries. This problem is easier to prevent than it is to treat, so it's never too late to try to slow the progress of this disease. When you prevent problems in the arteries of the legs, you also are taking steps to prevent the problem in the arteries in the heart. Such steps can prevent heart attack.

Medications

Medications can cause erectile dysfunction. Ask your doctor if any of your medications might be causing erection problems.

Hormones

Certain hormone problems can cause erectile dysfunction in addition to other illnesses. Your doctor can discover these when you have your check-up to be sure there are no specific hormonal problems causing your erectile dysfunction. These problems can often be treated, many times simply by taking a medication, as when the thyroid is underactive (hypothyroidism). These problems, if untreated, could lead to other complications and serious medical consequences, so the problem of erectile dysfunction might be a blessing in disguise, if it leads to their diagnosis.

Excessive or unusual stress

Stress can have a very strong impact on increasing erectile dysfunction. If you are in the midst of relationship problems with your wife or sexual partner, you're also at risk for erection problems. If you have major stress at work, financial problems creating stress, family members with problems, illness or death in the family, you may find that erections don't come as easy, don't last as long, or may fail altogether. Stress-related problems are often made worse by the idea that men should be able to have an erection at any time under almost any condition. This thinking ignores the fact that our emotions definitely affect erections.

Watch Out! Control hypertension and cholesterol to control peripheral vascular disease. If your blood pressure is above 145/85, or if your cholesterol is above 200, talk to your doctor.

What can you do about stress? Although we often can't control those events that cause stress—for example, we can't control illness in others or some financial problems—we can affect the way we handle the stress. Stress management can make a huge difference in how these problems affect our health and our lives. Lowering your stress may cure your erectile dysfunction.

Choosing Appropriate Therapy

You'll find there are a number of options for correcting erectile dysfunction. The easiest for many men is Viagra, the pill which can be taken before sexual activity.

After you have a medical check-up to find if there are any other contributing problems, your doctor can tell you which are your best choices. Viagra can be taken an hour before sexual activity and may be a good choice in your own situation, but it's important to get your doctor's approval first. Yohimbine is another oral medication which has been used by many for years, but has a low success rate. Still, since it is easy to take, if your doctor agrees, it may be worth a try.

The vacuum device (Erec-Aid) is successful in most patients, usually more than 80 percent. Some may find this device a little cumbersome at first, but it does work, and most patients who use it tend to continue using it over a long period of time. The fact that people continue to use it suggests that it is satisfactory as a solution for their particular problem.

Bright Idea
If your doctor agrees, add one aspirin and a vitamin E supplement (400 mg) daily to protect your heart.

Injections of medications into the penis (e.g., Caverject) are also popular because they work. The idea of injecting your penis is troublesome to many at first, but is usually quickly overcome as you learn more about the treatment. With this treatment, the medication is injected just before sexual activity. Cost is around $20 per injection, depending on the mixture of medication your urologist recommends.

Insertion of medication into the urethra (MUSE), instead of injecting the penis, is also effective for many. The medication is absorbed into the penis.

Other methods of treating impotence are discussed in Part III of this book. Read about them, then discuss these possibilities with your doctor.

When Your Doctor Says Surgery

While surgery seems like a very dramatic option to solve impotence, it does work. Surgery gives patients the comfort of knowing that there are almost always some options which will allow sexual activity and should be considered only after all the other options have been eliminated.

Surgery may be used to try to restore an arterial supply or to correct problems with the veins in the penis if one of these is found to be the major problem. However, these are not very common operations, and you should see a urologist who is experienced in the diagnosis of this problem and who has had success with the procedure.

The more common choice for surgery in erectile dysfunction is insertion of a penile implant, which is an artificial device that creates the erection. These are discussed in chapter 12.

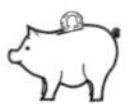

Moneysaver
Unlike other forms of impotence therapy, which range from $10 to $20 per treatment, the cost for a vacuum pump is around $400 to $500, a one-time cost.

Just the Facts

- Your doctor is used to questions about erectile dysfunction and has answers to solve this.
- There are known risk factors that can add to impotence, but most of these are controllable.
- Emotions definitely affect erections, so controlling stress is an important treatment method.

Chapter 16

GET THE SCOOP ON...

Why Viagra is considered a "lifestyle" drug ▪ Why women's groups oppose payment for Viagra ▪ How much some of the biggest insurers will pay for Viagra ▪ How to dispute a bill payment with your insurer

Who's Paying the Bill?

Before Viagra, millions of men (and their partners) suffered in silence because of the problem of erectile dysfunction. Since the advent of this medication, millions are calling their doctors for long-awaited prescriptions. Some urologists tell of getting a "hand stamp" saying "Viagra" because of cramped fingers from writing so many prescriptions!

The convenience of an oral medication that promises to give them back their sex lives is especially attractive to most men. For those who don't get relief from Viagra, at least the door has been opened for communication about the problem of impotence and other treatments that can work.

What Are Your Rights?

Because of the enthusiastic response to Viagra, more than two million prescriptions were written in the first three months. At $10 a pill, someone paid a large sum of money for this wonder drug—and in many cases, it was not the health insurance companies.

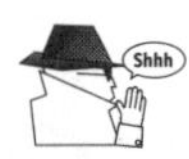

Unofficially... Before Viagra was released in spring l998, only about 10 percent of men with erectile dysfunction sought help.

Insurance companies have backed off from committing to pay for Viagra, and this has resulted in lawsuits from patients who feel they have the right to have sex, especially those with diseases like diabetes that have left them impotent.

Is it necessary?

This is the question insurance companies are asking the public. Is having sex necessary for your health? Does Viagra make you well? In some regards, this pill does help "make you well" as it treats impotence, which is extremely disabling for men and their partners. It also improves marital relationships that can help both men and women stay healthier. Studies have shown that couples who are happily married have less demand on the health-care system and stay healthier for longer periods of time. Researchers speculate that being happily married keeps our immune systems strong. Knowing that this social support is vital to wellness, and if Viagra helps men perform well sexually, then there must be a benefit to feeling good about yourself.

What the insurers claim

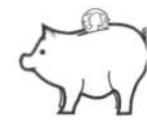

Moneysaver If you take Viagra, consider asking your doctor for the 100- mg tablets. Both 50- and 100-mg tablets cost about $10 each. With your doctor's permission, you can cut the 100-mg tablets in half and save money!

Most insurers do not agree with the above argument. The question they raise is basic and fundamental, that is, is treatment for diagnosed impotence medically necessary?

Seeing the skyrocketing popularity of Viagra, insurers were quick to put a halt on payment. Large companies like Oxford are refusing to pay for Viagra, yet already provide coverage for two invasive treatments—penile injections and a urethral suppository, which are comparable in cost. Both treatments are also not as convenient to use and are definitely not sought after by those with erectile dysfunction.

Lifestyle drugs

Viagra is not the first "lifestyle" drug that insurance companies have limited coverage for payments, but it is the one best publicized. A lifestyle drug is one that helps you feel better about yourself, yet it is not necessary to good health. They equate Viagra with other "quality of life" drugs such as:

- Retin-A - 900,000 people in America use Retin-A purely for wrinkles, instead of acne (which it was designed to combat).
- Five-million American men use hair-growing drugs like Rogaine or Propecia to avoid baldness.
- 14-million prescriptions have been written for diet drugs—most not for life-threatening obesity.

Of those who take diet pills, only 10 percent currently qualify for insurance coverage. Of those using Retin-A, about 65 percent are covered, but not for wrinkles. Almost none of those using drugs for baldness are covered.

Timesaver
If you check your insurance policy, most claim to provide coverage for all "prescription drugs" that are "medically necessary." Most exclude drugs that are "solely for convenience." Knowing this ahead of time will save you time in fighting a no-win situation.

Women's groups fight back

Insurance companies are not alone in opposing payment for Viagra. Women and their doctors have argued that covering Viagra, but not birth control methods, represents a sexual double standard. A 1994 report by the Alan Guttmacher Institute found that 97 percent of large group health insurance plans pay for prescription drugs. According to the Associated Press, however, only one-third of insurance companies cover birth control pills. Women's groups argue that if men are reimbursed for Viagra to make them sexually potent, women should be reimbursed for birth control pills to protect them from unwanted pregnancies.

Unofficially... As many as 73 percent of patients using anti-impotence drugs other than Viagra are reimbursed by health insurance, reports IMS, a private consulting group.

So Who's Going to Pay?

Doctors have prescribed Viagra for large numbers of patients (during the first few months after its release, doctors wrote more than 300,000 prescriptions per week). But Viagra has a drawback: it is expensive. In fact, all of the available treatments for impotence are expensive.

Since healthcare resources are limited, many health insurance companies have had to decide whether to cover the cost of Viagra and other treatments for erectile dysfunction.

The jury is still out

Some health plans are limiting the quantity of Viagra that they will cover. For example, Cigna will only cover the medication if the men have a "pre-existing documented condition of organic impotence, which is currently being treated by other medical means." Other companies require a special order from a physician to document that there is a medical cause of the erectile dysfunction. In other words, the insurance companies are using economics to regulate how sick you must be to receive help, and how frequently you can have sex. Doctors argue that they, and not the insurance company, should determine the appropriate supply of any medication.

During the clinical trials of Viagra, Pfizer provided the men in the study with eight pills a month. This amount was based on a 1994 University of Chicago study that concluded 41 percent of married couples have sex twice a week. Nonetheless, most health plans that cover Viagra only pay for six a month, and many health plans, including the Veterans' Administration hospitals, have at this time decided not to cover Viagra—yet you can opt for surgery to cure your impotence. This is usually covered by insurance plans, including Medicare, as are vacuum devices. The large insurers claim that providing the recommended six to 12 pills per month would be outrageously expensive, adding hundreds of millions of dollars to annual costs.

In fact, Kaiser Permanente, the nation's largest nonprofit health maintenance organization (HMO), which has 9.1-million members in 19 states, said the cost of covering Viagra would have exceeded $100 million a year. Aetna estimated that covering Viagra could add $50 million to its costs.

Watch Out!
If you use Viagra, be sure it is with your doctor's recommendation. This medication is now being promoted on the Internet, over 800 (toll free) lines, and in sex magazines. People who claim to be doctors are trying to sell prescriptions of Viagra to men across the globe—no questions asked.

Make a call

To find out if your health insurance covers Viagra or other treatments for erectile dysfunction, check with your doctor's office. Most doctors' offices deal with a variety of healthcare insurance plans, and each one's rules and policies change frequently. If you don't get a complete answer, call your health plan directly. Have the name and number of your policy or healthcare identification number ready. Be prepared to be switched to more than one person in the healthcare plan office, and be patient.

If your insurance carrier offers full or partial coverage, talk with your doctor so you can get the best possible treatment for your situation at the most reasonable cost. This may or may not be Viagra.

If the answer is no coverage, ask what you need to do to request an exception to allow coverage. Your healthcare plan administrator will tell you which forms and letters of medical necessity are required to be considered. Follow the rules. Be patient but persistent until you receive a clear answer. With all the new discussion on impotence, it is very likely that discussion and decision-making about the coverage of Viagra and other treatments for erectile dysfunction will also continue.

Watch Out!
Yes, that widely publicized herb may seem like it will help correct your erectile dysfunction, but is it effective or a fraud? Send for a copy of the National Consumer's League brochure on alternative medicine. Mail your request plus $1 for shipping and handling to: NCL, 1701 K Street, NW, Suite 1200, Washington, DC 20006, or phone (202) 835-3323.

Challenging Your Coverage

Once your insurance company refuses to pay for your impotence treatment, you may want to pursue this further. While you are doing this, write down any questions—no matter how trite they may seem—and ask your provider. For example, while your policy may cover treatment for hypertension, does it cover treatment for impotence if it is a side effect of the high blood pressure medication? Or, if your provider covers insulin for diabetes, does it cover treatment for erectile dysfunction as a result of the diabetes?

While you are reading your policy, find out how much is paid, if any, for impotence treatment, what the standard deductible is, and if this treatment must have a referral through your "gatekeeper." Many HMOs will not touch a treatment unless your gatekeeper or primary care doctor on the HMO's plan has referred you and unless the specialist you are referred to is listed on the plan.

Continue up the chain of authority with your insurance company until you are satisfied that you have spoken with someone who understands your policy. If you are not successful in obtaining coverage and you still feel as if you have a case to seek payment, document this, and go to small claims court.

Nevertheless, to avoid headaches and hassles regarding payment for services, check it out ahead of time to ensure the greatest success in getting your impotence treatment paid for without raising your blood pressure!

The Bottom Line

There are no easy answers about payment for impotence treatment. Some consumers in the United

States are waiting to see which companies cover Viagra and plan to change their policies to be sure of coverage. Those who have erectile dysfunction consider themselves seriously impaired and want to find ways to receive effective treatment. Yet money talks. Most insurers still feel that covering payments for Viagra is like covering cosmetic surgery and is simply not necessary. Conversely, insurers still pay for the older impotence treatments, such as penile implants, that involve the risk of invasive surgery, which can cost $15,000 to $20,000. Compared to Viagra, this cost is outrageous.

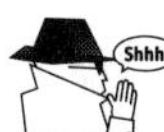

Unofficially... Recent nationwide polling shows that three- quarters of Americans favor insurance coverage of contraceptives, even if their premiums go up.

As a last resort, you might consider moving to England where insurance is available for erectile dysfunction. The policies pay for medical treatment for erectile dysfunction, which includes Viagra, as well as other treatments listed in this book. If no treatment works, the policy holder is paid £100,000 (about $150,000). The insurance company feels that Viagra will actually help them by having fewer payments of £100,000 for no effective treatment. And that's the bottom line!

Just the Facts

- Insurers are more likely to pay for penile injection therapy and urethral suppositories than for Viagra, even though the cost is about the same.
- In clinical trials, Pfizer provided study volunteers with eight Viagra pills a month, although most insurers that will reimburse for the drug are not authorizing that amount for consumers.
- If you have an HMO, you probably need a referral from your gatekeeper to see a urologist.

Chapter 17

GET THE SCOOP ON...

Why open communication is essential to solve this common problem ▪ The different alternatives available for counseling ▪ How counseling can help you gain coping skills to decrease stress ▪ The specific functions of a sex therapist

Working Together as a Couple

After you have thoroughly exhausted the medical resources to overcome impotence, your doctor may suggest that you work on this problem with your partner—together. In that regard, counseling or sex therapy may give great relief.

Finding workable answers is important as you seek to change your emotional response to erectile dysfunction. We list a host of alternative intervention strategies in this chapter. No matter which choices you make and carry out in your lifestyle, of paramount importance is accepting responsibility for your health.

Opening Doors of Communication

Everyone agrees that communication is essential in any relationship, especially when problems develop. When erectile dysfunction happens, it is a problem that affects not only the man who has it, but his partner as well, and in even the strongest partnerships,

Bright Idea
Keep in mind that psychological intervention is an accepted component for every man—not just the ones who have impotence problems.

the strain may be great enough to cause a disruption. The most common reaction is for the male partner to not talk about it. Another common reaction is to deny that there is a problem or to act as if he is no longer interested in sex.

Surveys have shown that most men would rather have hearing loss, cataracts, or hypertension than erectile dysfunction. The majority of women surveyed assumed their partner would not want them to initiate steps to treat erectile dysfunction. Ironically, almost half of the men surveyed would actually like it if their partner initiated the steps to get help. Is this a problem which communication might help?

Non-communication tends to drive a wedge between the couple. It can also spill over into other parts of their previously solid relationship as the female partner begins to wonder if she is no longer attractive enough or if the male partner is having another relationship.

The good news is that treatment is available, and Viagra has done a favor for all couples affected by erectile dysfunction by forcing the subject of impotence out into the open, which means treatments other than Viagra can also be discussed. In almost all cases, the problem can be solved, allowing couples to return to normal sexual activity. And with understanding of the entire relationship, you may be able to expand and actually increase your sexual enjoyment.

Starting Counseling

When your doctor or urologist says that you should see a psychologist or therapist, try to be open-minded about the possibility. If you really want to find an answer, it may be the fastest way to correct the problem, especially if your erectile dysfunction started during a period of severe stress.

Before you see this counselor, it's important to ask the urologist what may actually happen in therapy so you won't be surprised. You may find that a combination of counseling, as well as one of the other treatments discussed in this book, may present the best solution for solving your erectile problem.

Go alone initially

At first, you may be more comfortable one-on-one with the therapist. Through these initial conversations you will be able to restore your confidence by discovering what situations may be creating the erectile dysfunction and how you can resolve the problem. The problem of performance anxiety may be addressed in depth to further understand why it occurs and how to correct it.

Identifying stressors

The counselor will help you openly discuss the specific areas of stress that can contribute to erectile dysfunction, including stress from problems or failures at work, difficulties in relationships with your sexual partner, or other personal matters. Not only does stress make it difficult to handle everyday issues, it could definitely hinder any attempt you make at having a full erection.

Learning new coping skills

The role of psychological counseling in helping to overcome impotence can help you to develop appropriate coping strategies for dealing with issues of high stress in your life.

Psychological intervention can give you coping methods that you can use either within or outside other treatment programs. In most cases, it is important that the person providing these services is familiar with male sexual problems.

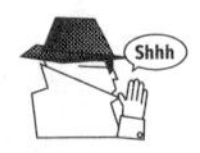

Unofficially... The sexual problems people relate most frequently have to do with inhibitions and guilt, performance anxiety, erotic boredom, and blind acceptance of sexual misinformation or myths. These four problems collectively account for more than 80 percent of the sexual dissatisfaction in modern America.

Available options

Some of the options for counseling include:

- *Individual counseling.* This is a one-on-one session with a therapist where you can address your personal problem areas. These sessions may include specific help with alleviating depression, anxiety, or stress, along with other issues such as work-related situations or relationship difficulties.

- *Marriage counseling.* Erectile problems obviously extend beyond you to also affect your spouse. Therefore, it is often helpful for both husband and wife (or partner) to understand and accept the problem, as well as the possible impact it may have on the relationship. While your spouse or partner may have the best of intentions, without specific guidance, they sometimes make things worse. This counseling may open the door to better communication between your spouse and you and allow you to openly discuss the problem and see possible solutions.

- *Group counseling.* There is no one who can better understand you than another person with the same problem. Group sessions led by trained sex therapists allow for the sharing of feelings, as well as the development of effective coping strategies. The exchange of ideas at group sessions is often the most productive way to revamp your thought processes and get over stumbling blocks like "performance anxiety."

- *Support groups.* In a support group, you can share your feelings with others suffering from similar sexual problems. Members of support groups can also receive comfort and encouragement from each other. The latest available treatments can be discussed and members can give coping suggestions while affirming the positive experiences of each other. The realization that "someone else knows what I am going through" is helpful as people share their struggles. Support groups are not meant to be professional therapy groups. Those who would benefit from standard psychological or psychiatric intervention should seek professional treatment to fit their needs, though it is not uncommon for people to simultaneously see a therapist and to belong to a support group.

Sex Therapy Is Effective Treatment

Sex therapy may be a treatment you should consider to help in communication and understanding. A sex therapist is also a counselor, but one who is trained in the professional and ethical management of sexual function and problems related to sexual expression.

Many people consider the idea of sex therapy "dirty" or something not to be talked about. Most people have not discussed the details of their sexual function, and most men with erectile dysfunction would not discuss it with their wife, lover, or their best friend. Finding a safe, confidential, and knowledgeable expert may be a way for you to learn more about the causes of and treatments for erectile dysfunction. At the same time, you may want to explore other questions about your sexual function as an individual or as a couple.

Bright Idea
Some professional associations that give specialists a standard for level of care include The American Association for Marriage and Family Therapy, and The American Association of Sex Educators, Counselors and Therapists. If your specialist is a member of one or both of these groups, then you have some measure of their qualifications.

An identity problem

Sex therapists understand that for many individuals, sexual function is closely tied to their identity. Sexual problems can therefore lead to loss of self-esteem. And dissatisfaction with a sexual relationship may lead to negative feelings that can be destructive to the entire relationship, even causing an end to the relationship.

Sex therapists help men and women understand and treat almost all aspects of sexuality. This may include problems with erectile dysfunction, other problems of impotence, or sexual problems brought on by physical disabilities, illnesses, or surgery. You should feel comfortable with your sex therapist, who should be skilled in all areas of sexual counseling.

Seek qualified professionals

Ask your doctor or urologist for the names of sex therapists in your area who they trust and who other professionals have used with success. Be sure you choose a well-trained specialist.

With a qualified sex therapist, you'll find confidential counseling that will address your specific problems in detail and in a non-judgmental way. You'll also be guided to those specialists needed to help resolve your problem, whether it be a physician such as a urologist, an internal medicine specialist, or other healthcare professional.

Professional referrals

For helpful referrals or references, contact the following:

- **American Association for Marriage and Family Therapy**: 1100 17th Street, NW, 10th Floor
  Washington, DC 20036
  Telephone (202) 452-0109

- **American Association of Sex Educators, Counselors and Therapists:** P.O. Box 238
  Mt. Vernon, IA 52314
- **American Academy of Clinical Sexologists**:
  1929 18th Street, NW, Suite 1166
  Washington, DC 20009
  Telephone (202) 462-2122

Further reading

If you would rather read more about sex therapy and how it may help your relationship, consider one of the following books:

- *From the Files of a Sex Therapist: Bedroom Secrets Teach Keys to Success,* by Carole Altman, Lifetime Books; ISBN: 0811908747
- *Bridging Separate Gender Worlds: Why Men and Women Clash and How Therapists Can Bring Them Together,* by Carol L. Philpot, Gary R. Brooks, Don-David Lusterman, American Psychological Association; ISBN: 155798381X
- *Integrative Couple Therapy: Promoting Acceptance and Change,* by Neil S. Jacobson, Andrew Christensen, W. W. Norton & Company; ISBN: 0393702316
- *Passion Play: Ancient Secrets for a Lifetime of Health and Happiness Through Sensational Sex,* by Felice Dunas, Philip Goldberg, Putnam Publishing Group; ISBN: 1573220760
- *Sacred Relationships; The Psychospiritual Path to Love, Intimacy and Happiness,* by Donna L., Dr. Boone, R. Michael, Dr. McDonald, Benthall Hall Publishers; ISBN: 0965884104

- *Seven Weeks to Better Sex,* by Domeena Renshaw, Pam Brick, Dell Books (Paperbacks); ISBN: 0440507529
- *You Can Be Your Own Sex Therapist: A Systematized Behavioral Approach to Enhancing Your Sensual Pleasures, Improving Your Sexual Enjoyment,* by Carole Altman, Casper Publishing; ISBN: 0965752798

Seek Answers

We've introduced you to a wealth of information regarding erectile dysfunction. Hopefully, at this time, you are not feeling so alone and frightened. Perhaps you now understand that this condition is extremely common, as well as treatable.

Talk to your doctor. Communicate with your spouse or partner. Reduce your risk factors for serious diseases, and seek treatments that really work for you.

The answers are out there—you just have to ask the right questions!

Just the Facts

- Viagra has opened the door for impotence to be discussed openly.
- Counseling can be done individually, as a couple, or within the support of a group of people with similar concerns.
- A sex therapist is someone who helps to explore sexual problems and function.

Appendix A

Recommended Reading List

Abrahams, Allen E., and Steven Morganstern.
Overcoming Impotence: A Doctor's Proven Guide to Regaining Sexual Vitality. (Prentice Hall)

Beck, Dr. N.
Impotence Assist: The Causes, Treatments, and Prevention of Weak Erections (Impotence) and Premature Ejaculation.
(Internet Language Company)

Butler, Robert N., Myrna I. Lewis, and Trey Sunderland.
Aging & Mental Health: Positive Psychosocial & Biomedical Approaches. (Prentice Hall)

Chase, Jim, and Peter Dorsen.
Dr. D's Handbook for Men over 40: A Guide to Health, Fitness, Living, and Loving in the Prime of Life.
(Chronimed Publishing)

Dzurinko, Mary, and Diane Kaschak Newman.
The Urinary Incontinence Sourcebook.
(Contemporary Books, Inc.)

George, Stephen C.
Fight Fat: A Total Lifestyle Program for Men to Stay Slim and Healthy. (Rodale Press)

Hopkins, Virginia L., Earl L. Mindell, and Earl R. Mindell.
Dr. Earl Mindell's What You Should Know About Natural Health for Men. (Keats Publishing)

Lafavore, Michael.
Men's Health Today. (Rodale Press)

Men's Health Today 1998: The Most Important, Current Tips and Tools for Healthy, Strong Living.
Edited by Michael Lafavore. (Rodale Press)

Mobley, David, and Steven K. Wilson.
Impotence Is Reversible—Forever. (Swan Publishing Co.)

Penn, Robert E.
The Gay Men's Wellness Guide: The National Lesbian and Gay Health Association's Complete Book of Physical, Emotional, and Mental Health and Well-being.
(Henry Holt and Company)

Somer, Elizabeth.
Age-Proof Your Body: Your Complete Guide to Lifelong Vitality. (William Morrow & Co.)

Steidle, Christopher P.
The Impotence Sourcebook. (Lowell House)

Yosh, Taguchi, M.D.
Private Parts: An Owner's Guide to the Male Anatomy.

Appendix B

Important Statistics

We now know that the majority of cases (80 percent of all cases of impotency) are caused by *physical problems.*

Before the impotence pill Viagra was released, most men were treated by external vacuum therapy, penile injection, implant surgery, or intra-urethral pellet implantation. Estimates of treatment prescribed annually include 150,000 vacuum devices, 700,000 penile injections, and 21,000 penile implants.

According to a 1992 National Institutes of Health conference study of the problem, impotence includes anything from "inability to get an erection" to "unsatisfactory sexual performance."

Medications cause 25 percent of all cases of impotence.

Some type of erectile dysfunction affects more than 50 percent of men age 40 to 70 worldwide.

This breaks down to one out of every 10 males in the United States, yet only about 5 percent of these men seek treatment.

Research shows that up to 39 percent of men will have some problem with erection by the time they reach age 40.

This number dramatically increases as men age. By age 70, about two-thirds of all men will suffer from some type of erection problem.

Endocrine or glandular disorders cause hormonal problems that account for 3 percent of erectile failure.

Sexual Activity

Some researchers have found that more than 70 percent of couples are still sexually active at age 68. Others have reported that more than 80 percent of couples over age 60 are sexually active, and at least half have regular sexual activity.

According to Masters and Johnson, at least 25 to 30 percent of people in their 60s have intercourse at least weekly.

A study of Swedish men found that 83 percent of men age 50 to 80 said sex was very important to them.

Although erection problems increase with age, half of men age 70 to 80 years are still sexually active.

A study of American men found that 80 percent of men age 51 to 64 had sex weekly.

Another study of Americans found that 80 percent of men over age 69 are still sexually active.

Some researchers have found that although the frequency of sex decreases over time, 75 percent of some groups over age 60 claimed that sex was the same or better at that age than when they were younger.

Men's Health

Studies show that one out of every 10 men in the United States has erectile dysfunction at some time; it is usually not a psychological problem and is almost always treatable.

According to a recent survey conducted by *Men's Health* magazine and CNN, one-third of American men have not had a check-up in the past year. Nine-million men haven't seen a doctor in five years.

Annually, men make 150-million fewer trips to doctors than women.

According to a 1990 American Medical Association study, men don't go to the doctor because of fear, denial, embarrassment, and threatened masculinity.

One in nine men will be diagnosed with prostate cancer, yet few will have the easy and painless digital rectal exam and prostate-specific antigen (PSA) blood test that could detect it.

Testicular cancer is 95 percent curable if caught early enough.

Men are at greater risk of stress-related illnesses than women, yet only 20 percent of those attending the typical stress-management program are men.

Men are 30 percent more likely than women to have a stroke.

One out of three male strokes occur before age 65.

Every year, over 50,000 men die of emphysema, one of the most preventable diseases.

It has been estimated that more than 3 million men are in the early stages of type 2 diabetes, a disease with major complications, and don't know it. Nearly one-third of men in the United States are overweight.

Almost four times as many men as women suffer heart attacks before age 65. Some 27 percent of men die within one year of suffering a heart attack. Research shows that more than 40 percent of men have erectile dysfunction after suffering a heart attack.

Peyronie's disease is a relatively rare condition in which an inflammation within the penis causes scarring. This leads to a curvature, causing painful erections. The bending of the penis can also interfere with sexual activity.

Despite advances in medical technology and research, the life expectancy of men continues to be seven years less than that of women.

Prostate Disease and Prostate Cancer

The first changes in the prostate occur in most men by age 35 with some increase in size.

Over half of men have symptoms of prostate enlargement by age 69, and almost every man develops the condition eventually.

Commonly, men over the age of 50 will suffer from benign prostatic hyperplasia (BPH).

More than 50 percent of men over the age of 60 have benign prostatic hypertrophy and approximately 20 to 25 percent of those require treatment. Prostate cancer is the second leading cause of death from cancer in males in the United States.

Prostate cancer is especially common in males over 60 and accounts for over 40,000 deaths annually.

Approximately 100,000 men a year are diagnosed with prostate cancer and more than an estimated 30,000 will die from the disease in 1998.

Prostate cancer is rare in men younger than age 40, but the incidence of this cancer increases with age, especially after the age of 55. Eighty percent of all cases of prostate cancer occur in men who are 65 or older. The good news is that this type of cancer can be controlled if detected early.

The incidence of prostate cancer is 50 percent higher in African-Americans than in whites.

If you have a family member with prostate cancer, you may be at higher than average risk, especially if they were affected in their 40s or 50s.

The relative risk in men with one affected immediate family member has been estimated as twice that of an individual without a family history of prostate cancer. If there are two affected relatives, the risk is approximately five times greater than normal.

The death rate from prostate cancer has increased by 25 percent since 1971.

An estimated 334,500 new cases will be diagnosed in 1998.

One in five men in the United States will develop prostate cancer.

Currently about 70 percent of all prostate cancer patients are alive five years after diagnosis, and half of these men had their cancer detected early.

An estimated 3.6-million men have Type 2 diabetes and don't know it.

Diabetes affects more than 12-million Americans, and about 4 percent of all women and 2 percent of men in the United States become diabetic.

About half of all diabetic men have problems with erection, which can be caused by damage to the nerves that supply the penis and erection, or from atherosclerosis, which is more common in diabetics. Diabetes often creeps up on you, as it has for an estimated 100-million people afflicted worldwide.

Because the initial symptoms (fatigue, frequent urination) of diabetes are usually mild, half of the millions of Americans with diabetes do not realize they have it.

Obesity and overweight is a health problem that affects 97-million American adults, or 55 percent of the population.

Scientific studies reveal that maintaining blood sugar levels (near normal) may reduce the risk of complications by 50 to 90 percent.

Research shows that aggressive treatment with diet, physical activity, and new medicines can prevent or delay much of the illness or death caused by diabetes.

Minorities are at high risk for diabetes, experiencing complications that show up in high rates of eye disease, kidney disease, amputations, and premature deaths.

An estimated 16-million Americans have diabetes, including 5.4 million not yet diagnosed.

The prevalence of diabetes is rising as the U.S. population ages and as more Americans become obese.

Diabetes is the leading cause of adult blindness, end-stage kidney disease, and amputations of the foot and leg.

About one-half of all men with diabetes suffer with impotence.

People with diabetes have an increased risk of heart disease and stroke.

Aging and Sexual Health

Hormonal problems, as a result of endocrine or glandular disorders, account for only 3 percent of erectile failure. The testicles may produce too little testosterone, leading to a decrease in desire and sexual dysfunction.

Men experience a subtle testosterone loss (about 1 percent per year after age 40, or 30-percent decline by age 70).

After age 40, low testosterone levels can be common in men. Even though testosterone levels become lower normally, they still may be in the "normal" range.

Appendix C

Available Internet Sites

National Automobile Dealers Association
www.nada.com

American College of Gastroenterology
Drug, health, product, and health information pertaining to medical treatment of disorders of the gastrointestinal (GI) tract.
www.acg.gi.org

American College of Rheumatology
Drug, health, product, and health information pertaining to arthritis and arthritis-related diseases.
www.rheumatology.org

American Diabetes Association
Diabetes information, research, Internet resources, and more.
www.diabetes.org/default.htm

American Heart Association
www.amhrt.org/

American Board of Sexology
Listing of board certified sex therapists (search by state).
www.sexologist.org

American Cancer Society
www.cancer.org

Ayurvedic Health Center
www.ayurvedic.org

Ayurvedic Foundation
www.ayur.com

Ayurvedic Newsgroup
www.alt.health.ayurveda

Cancer Information Service National Cancer Institute
www.nci.nih.gov/

Cancer Care, Inc.
Cancer Resource
www.cancercareinc.org/

Chiropractic Online
www.amerchiro.org/

Diabetes Information Sites
www.ndep.nih.gov
www.cdc.gov/diabetes

HEALTH CARE
www.columbia.net

HealthTouchKidney
Urologic and sexual problems
www.healthtouch.com

National Heart, Lung, and Blood Institute Information Center
Supporting research and training in the prevention, diagnosis, and treatment of cardiovascular diseases.
www.nhlbi.nih.gov/nhlbi/nhlbi.htm

National Institute of Mental Health (NIMH)
Some of the subjects covered are: Alzheimer's disease, AIDS, anxiety and panic disorder, depression, bipolar disorder, schizophrenia, paranoia, obsessive-compulsive disorder, attention-deficit hyperactivity disorder, anorexia nervosa and bulimia, phobias, suicide, stress, family mental health, mental health of the aging, minority and special populations, and attitudes toward mental illness.
www.nimh.nih.gov

National Institute of Neurological Disorders and Stroke (NINDS)
National Institutes of Health
This institute supports and conducts research on brain and nervous system disorders.
www.ninds.nih.gov

National Mental Health Association (NMHA)
NMHA is a voluntary charitable organization with more than 80 years of success in addressing the mental health needs of our communities, states, and nation.
www.nmha.org

National Sleep Foundation
The National Sleep Foundation provides free brochures on sleep, drowsy driving and sleep disorders, regional listings of accredited sleep centers, and other public education materials.
www.sleepfoundation.org
e-mail: natsleep@erols.com

Weight-Control Information Network
A service of the National Institute of Diabetes and Digestive and Kidney Diseases, part of the National Institutes of Health. Responds to requests for information. Develops communications strategies to encourage individuals to achieve and maintain a healthy weight.
www.niddk.nih.gov/health/nutrit/win.htm

National Clearinghouse for Alcohol and Drug Information
A free service; clearinghouse containing the most comprehensive collection of scientific and consumer-oriented

information on alcohol and other drugs in the U.S.
www.health.org

Food and Drug Administration—AIDS Information
Consumer information on AIDS.
www.fda.gov

Centers for Disease Control and Prevention—AIDS
The CDC National AIDS Clearinghouse serves as the principal point of HIV/AIDS information collection and dissemination for the Centers for Disease Control and Prevention and the Public Health Service. All of the CDC NAC's services are designed to facilitate the sharing of resources and information about education and prevention, published materials, and research findings as well as news about AIDS-related trends.
www.cdc.gov

Impotence Institute of America and Impotence
Information on impotence.
www.urologyinstitute.org

Impotence Resource Center
Current literature and information on men's sexuality and health.
www.impotence.org/info.htm

Sexual Function Health Council
Brochures on impotence.
www.iiem.org

Thrive Online
Great site for current information on men's health, sexuality, diseases, and more.
www.thriveonline.com/

Doctor's Guide Information and resources on diabetes.
www.pslgroup.com/DIABETES.htm

Diabetes.com
Support groups, risk factors, prevention, newly diagnosed, and more.
www.diabetes.com

Healthy World Online
www.healthy.net

Heart Information Network
Heart disease information.
www.heartinfo.org

Herbal Research
www.herbs.org/index.html

Herbal Providers
www.frontierherb.com/homepage.html

Herbal Resources
www.herbnet.com/

Impotence site
www.impotence.org/

Impotence site
www2.impotent.com/caverject/

InterNational Council on Infertility Information Dissemination
The INCIID Hot Links list now contains more than 150 infertility, pregnancy loss, and alternative family building links.

www.inciid.org
e-mail: INCIIDinfo@inciid.org

Internet Mental Health
www.mentalhealth.com

Journal of Urology Highlights
Highlights from the Journal of Urology.
www.auanet.org

Mayo Health Oasis
General medical information site.
www.mayohealth.org

Mediconsult
This Web site has information on many subjects such as PDQ for patients, prostate cancer, benign prostatic hypertrophy support groups, infertility support groups, prostate cancer support groups, men's health, stress, depression, erectile dysfunction, and more.
www.mediconsult.com

Mental Health Net
www.cmhc.com

National Institutes of Health
www.nih.gov

Doctor's Guide
Information and resources on diabetes.
www.pslgroup.com/DIABETES.htm

COHIS: HealthSource; Diabetes
A list of diabetes organizations and foundations on the Web; Online Journals Current and important information from online magazines on diabetes; Online Bookstores Browse and order publications on diabetes from the comfort of your computer; Diabetes, Risk Test—Could you have diabetes and not know it?
web.bu.edu/COHIS/hsource/diabetes.htm

National Library of Medicine
www.nlm.nih.gov/

Office of Alternative Medicine
altmed.od.nih.gov/oam/

Prostate problems
rattler.cameron.edu/prostate/prostate.html

Prostatitis
www.msn.fullfeed.com/~prosfnd/

Sympatico
Various Web sites having to do with impotence, sexuality, education, and more.
www.sympatico.ca/

Johns Hopkins Health Information
Kidney and urologic site.
www.intelihealth.com

The American Urological Association
Information resource on urologic diseases.
www.auanet.org

The Male Health Center
Men's health resource.
www.malehealthcenter.com

The National Institute of Diabetes and Digestive and Kidney Diseases
Diabetes, digestive, and kidney resource site.
www.niddk.nih.gov/NIDDK_HomePage.html

Urology News
Urology News Online is a bimonthly review of current literature in urology and related fields. Each issue of Urology News Online will offer lead articles and features on areas of current interest, important conference reviews, product information, and more. Links to related sites are also included.
www.uronews.com/

US TOO International, Inc.
Prostate cancer survivors and families. Education and support through an international network of support groups, literature, newsletters, and toll-free hotline.
1-800-808-7866
www.ustoo.com

Appendix D

Recommended Resources

AARP
American Association of Retired Persons
601 E. Street, N.W.
Washington, DC 20049

Write to the Research Information Group, c/o AARP. You will receive an order form listing available brochures. Allow 4 to 6 weeks. This organization should be able to point you in the right direction on almost any issue dealing with aging, as well as offer you numerous booklets on aging.

Acupressure-Acupuncture Institute, Inc.
10506 N. Kendall Drive
Miami, Florida 33176
Phone: 305-595-9500
Fax: 305-595-2622

Acupressure Institute
1533 Shattuck Ave.
Berkeley, CA 94709
Toll free: 800-442-2232 (outside California)
Phone: 510-845-1059 (inside California)

Advil Forum on Healthcare
1500 Broadway, 26th Floor
New York, NY 10036

Ask for a brochure on pain relief for back pain or arthritis.

Aids for Arthritis
3 Little Knoll Court
Medford, NJ 08055
609-654-6918

AIDS Hotline
800-342-AIDS
Spanish: 800-344-7432
Deaf: 800-243-7889

Alexander Technique
1692 Massachusetts Ave., 3rd Floor
Cambridge, MA 02138
Phone: 617-497-2242
Fax: 617-497-2615

Alliance for Alternatives in Healthcare, Inc.
P.O. Box 6279
Thousand Oaks, CA 91359
Phone: 805-494-7818
Fax: 805-494-8528

Alliance for Natural Health
P.O. Box 4035
Hammond, IN 46324
Phone: 708-974-9373
Fax: 708-974-6002

Alternative Health Insurance Services, Inc.
P.O. Box 6279
Thousand Oaks, CA 91359-6279
Toll free: 800-966-8467
Fax: 805-379-1580

The Alternative Medicine Connection
Healthsavers Press, P.O. Box 683
Herndon, VA 22070
703-471-8465

Alternative Medicine Digest
Toll free: 800-333-HEAL
Web site: www.alternativemedicine.com

Alternative Medicine Political Action Committee, Inc.
1718 M. St., #205
Washington, DC 20036

Alternative Therapies Associations
Life Extension Foundation
P.O. Box 229120
Hollywood, FL 33022-9120
800-841-5433

American Academy of Allergy, Asthma & Immunology (AAAAI)
611 East Wells St.
Milwaukee, WI 53202
Phone: 414-272-6071
Toll free: 800-822-ASMA

American Academy of Clinical Sexologists
202-464-2122

American Academy of Environmental Physicians
913-642-6062

American Academy of Medical Acupuncture
5820 Wilshire Blvd., Suite 500
Los Angeles, CA 90036
Phone: 213-937-5514
Toll free: 800-521-AAMA
Web site: www.medicalacupuncture.org

American Academy of Osteopathy (AAO)
3500 DePauw Blvd., Suite 1080
Indianapolis, IN 46268
317-879-1881

American Academy of Pediatrics
Department of Publications
P.O. Box 927
Elk Grove Village, IL 60007

American Allergy Association
P.O. Box 7273
Menlo Park, CA 94026

American Association of Acupuncture and Bio-Energetic Medicine (AAABEM)
2512 Manoa Road
Honolulu, HI 96822
Phone: 808-946-2069
Fax: 808-946-0378

American Association of Acupuncture and Oriental Medicine
4101 Lake Boone Trail, Suite 201
Raleigh, NC 27607
919-787-5181

American Association of Alternative Medicine, Inc.
1000 Rutherford Road
Landrum, SC 29356

American Association of Certified Allergists (AACA)
85 West Algonquin Road, Suite 550
Arlington Heights, IL 60005

American Association of Kidney Patients
100 S. Ashley Drive, Suite 280
Tampa, FL 33602
800-749-2257

The American Association of Naturopathic Physicians
601 Valley Street, Suite 105
Seattle, WA 98109
Phone: 206-298-0126
Fax: 206-209-0129

American Association of Oriental Medicine
433 Front Street
Catasauqua, PA 18032
Phone: 610-266-1433
Fax: 610-264-2768

American Association of Respiratory Care
11030 Ables Lane
Dallas, TX 75229-4593

American Botanical Council
P.O. Box 2016601
Austin, TX 78720
American Cancer Society
1599 Clifton Rd., N.E.
Atlanta, GA 30329
800-ACS-2345

American Chiropractic Association (ACA)
1701 Claredon Blvd.
Arlington, VA 22209
Phone: 703-276-8800
Toll free: 800-986-4636

American Chronic Pain Association
P.O. Box 850
Rocklin, CA 95677
Phone: 916-632-0922
Fax: 916-632-3208

American College for Advancement in Medicine
23121 Verdugo Drive, Suite 204
Laguna Hills, CA 92653

American College of Allergy and Immunology
800 E. Northwest Highway, Suite 1080
Palatine, IL 60067
Phone: 708-359-2800
Toll free: 800-842-7777

American College of Gastroenterology
4900 B South 31st Street
Arlington, VA 22206-1656
703-820-7400

American College of Rheumatology
60 Executive Park South, Suite 150
Atlanta, GA 30329
404-633-3777

American Dance Therapy Association
2000 Century Plaza, Suite 108
Columbia, MD 21044-3263
410-997-4040

American Diabetes Association
1660 Duke St.
P.O. Box 25757
Alexandria, VA 22314
800-232-3472

American Dietetic Association
Toll-free Nutritional Hotline: 800-366-1655

American Heart Association
7272 Greenville Ave.
Dallas, TX 75231-4596
214-373-6300

American Herbal Pharmacopeia™
Box 5159
Santa Cruz, CA 95063
Phone: 408-461-6317
Fax: 408-438-7410

American Herbal Products Association
P.O. Box 2410
Austin, TX 78768
512-320-8555

The American Herbalists Guild
P.O. Box 1683
Sequel, CA 95073

American Holistic Medical Association
4101 Lake Boone Trail, Suite 201
Raleigh, NC 27607

American Lung Association
432 Park Ave., S.
New York, NY 10016
800-LUNG-USA

American Massage Therapy Association
820 Davis Street, Suite 100
Evanston, IL 60201-4444
Phone: 847-864-0123
Fax: 847-864-1178
Web site: www.amtamassage.org

American Natural Hygiene Society
P.O. Box 30630
Tampa, FL 33630
813-855-6607

American Osteopathic Association
142 East Ontario Street
Chicago, IL 60611
800-621-1773

American Preventive Medical Association
459 Walker Road
Great Falls, VA 22066
703-759-0662

American Psychiatric Association
202-682-6000

The American Psychological Association
202-336-5700

American School of Ayurvedic Sciences
10025 N.E. 4th Street
Bellevue, WA 98004
206-453-8022

American Self-Help Clearinghouse
St. Clare's-Riverside Medical Center
Pocono Road
Denville, NJ 07834
201-625-7101

American Sleep Disorders Association
1610 14th Street N.W., Suite 300
Rochester, MN 55901

American Speech-Language-Hearing Association
National Office
10801 Rockville Pike
Rockville, MD 20852
Phone: 301-897-5700
Fax: 301-571-0457

Anxiety Disorders Association of America
6000 Executive Blvd., Suite 513
Rockville, MD 20852
301-231-9350

Area Agency on Aging
U.S. Department of Health and Human Services
Dept. BHG
Independence Avenue, S.W.
Washington, DC 20201

Arthritis Foundation
1314 Spring Street
Atlanta, GA 30309
Toll free: 800-283-7800

Arthritis Society
250 Floor Street East, Suite 901
Toronto, Ontario,
Canada M4W 3P2
416-967-1414

Associated Bodywork and Massage Professionals
Toll free: 800-458-2267
Web site: www.abmp.com

Association of Applied Psychophysiology and Biofeedback
10200 West 44th Ave., Suite 304
Wheat Ridge, CO 80033-2840
303-422-8436

Asthma & Allergy Foundation of America (AAFA)
1125 15th Street N.W., Suite 502
Washington, DC 20005
Toll free: 800-624-0044 or 800-7-ASTHMA

Asthma Zero Mortality Coalition
800-777-4350

Austin Nutritional Research
4815 West Braker Lane
Building 502, Suite 180
Austin, TX 78759
Phone: 512-267-7644
Fax: 512-267-4448
Web site: www.realtime.net/anr/catalog.html

Ayurvedic Foundations
1550 East 3300 South
Salt Lake City, UT 84106
801-466-8324

Ayurvedic Institute
11311 Menaul N.E., Suite A
Albuquerque, NM 87112
595-291-9698

Back Pain Association of America
P.O. Box 135
Pasadena, MD 21122
Phone: 410-255-3633
Fax: 410-255-7338

Biofeedback Certification Institute of America
10200 W. 44th Avenue, Suite 304
Wheat Ridge, CO 80033
Phone: 303-420-2902
Web site: www.bcia.org

Cancer Care, Inc.
The Prostate Cancer Education Council
800-813-HOPE
Provides resource information, referrals, counseling, and support to cancer patients and their families.

Centers for Disease Control and Prevention—
AIDS Information
P.O. Box 6003
Rockville, MD 20849-6003

Clearinghouse of Disability
U.S. Department of Education
Office of Special Education and Rehab. Services
Switzer Building, Room 3132
Washington, DC 20202-2524
202-708-5366

Consumer Information Center
S. James
P.O. Box 100
Pueblo, CO 81002
719-948-9724

Disabled Sportsman
P.O. Box 5496
Roanoke, VA 24012

Enzymatic Therapy
825 Challenger Drive
Green Bay, WI 54311-8328
920-469-4419

Fernwood Herb Farms
P.O. Box 332
Fernwood, ID 83830

Fibromyalgia Association
P.O. Box 21988
Columbus, OH 43221-0988
Phone: 614-457-4222
Fax: 614-457-2729

Fibromyalgia Network
5700 Stockdale Highway, Suite 100
Bakersfield, CA 93309
805-631-1950

Food Allergy Network
10400 Eaton Place, Suite 107
Fairfax, VA 22030-2208
703-691-3179

Food and Drug Administration—
AIDS Information
5600 Fishers Lane
Rockville, MD 20857
Consumer Information Line: 301-827-4420

Group Health Cooperative
Phone: 206-901-4636
Toll free: 888-901-4636
Fax: 206-901-4612

Group Health Insurance Services
Toll free: 800-358-8815 (individual)
Toll free: 800-542-6312
Two Embarcadaro Center
Suite 600
San Francisco, CA 94111
415-248-2700

Help for Incontinent People
P.O. Box 544
Union, SC 29379

The Herb Growing and Marketing Network
P.O. Box 245
Silver Spring, PA 17575
717-393-3295

Herb Research Foundation
1007 Pearl Street, Suite 200
Boulder, CO 80302
Phone: 303-449-2265
Fax: 303-449-7849

Herb Society of America
9019 Kirtland-Chardon Road
Kirtland, OH 44094
Phone: 216-256-0514
Fax: 216-256-0541

Herbal Valley
1664 North Cedar Street, #85
Laramie, WY 82072
Toll free: 800-644-2482

Homeocare
ELS International, Inc.
P.O. Box 630115
Riverdale, NY 10463
Phone: 888-HOMEOCARE
Fax: 718-796-7292

Homeopathic Educational Services
2124 Kittredge Street
Berkeley, CA 94704
Phone: 800-359-9051
Fax: 510-649-1955

Hoosier Herbal Remedies
6816 Pebblebrook Court
Brownsburg, IN 46112
317-852-4997

Impotence Information Center
(Centro de Información sobre la Impotencia)
P.O. Box 9
Minneapolis, MN 55440
800-843-4315

Impotence Institute of America (IIA)
(Instituto Americano de La Impotencia)
10400 Patuxent Parkway, Suite 485
Columbia, MD 21044-3502
800-669-1603

Impotence Resource Center
800-433-4215

Imprints Magazine
Birth and Life Bookstore
7001 Alonzo Avenue, N.W.
P.O. Box 70625
Seattle, WA 98107

International Association of Infant Massage
1720 Willow Creek Circle, Suite 516
Eugene, OR 97402
Toll free: 800-248-5432

International Chiropractors Association (ICA)
1110 N. Glebe Road, Suite 1000
Arlington, VA 22201
Phone: 703-528-5000
Toll free: 800-423-4690

International Foundation for Homeopathy
2366 Eastlake Avenue East, Suite 325
Seattle, WA 98102
206-776-4146

International Herb Association
P.O. Box 317
Mundelein, IL 60060-0317
Phone: 847-949-4372
Fax: 847-949-5896

International Massage Association
Phone: 202-387-6555
Web site: www.imagroup.com

International Society for Orthomolecular Medicine
16 Florence Ave.
Toronto, Ontario,
Canada M2N 1E9
416-733-2117

Internet Mental Health
601 West Broadway, Suite 902
Vancouver, B.C.,
Canada
V5Z 4C2

Journal of Herbs, Spices & Medicinal Plants
Haworth Press, Inc.
10 Alice St.
Binghamton, NY 13904-1580

Journal of Naturopathic Medicine
10 Morgan Avenue
Norwalk, CT 06851

Kaiser Foundation Health Plan
510-596-1120

Macrobiotic Center
61 E. 81st Street, Suite 65
New York, NY 10028
212-505-1010

Macrobiotic products
Kushi Cuisine
Toll free: 800-490-0044

Managing Medications
Dept. S
P.O. Box 15329
Stanford, CT 06901

Manitoba Lung Association
629 McDermot Ave.
Winnipeg, Manitoba,
Canada R3A 1P6
204-774-5501

National Arthritis & Musculoskeletal & Skin Diseases Information Clearinghouse
One AMS Circle
Bethesda, MD 20892-3675
301-495-4484

National Association for Holistic Aromatherapy
P.O. Box 17622
Boulder, CO 80308-0622
303-258-3791

National Association of Area Agencies on Aging
1112 16th Street N.W., Suite 100
Washington, DC 20036
Check for the agency in your town or call 800-555-1212 to get the number of the nearest agency.

The National Association of Certified Natural Health Professionals
810 S. Buffalo Street
Warsaw, IN 46580

The National Association of Diabetes Educators
800-832-6874

National Association of Managed Care Professionals (NAMCP)
4435 Waterfront Drive, Suite 101
Glen Allen, VA 23060
Toll free: 800-722-0376

The National Association of Social Workers
202-408-8600

National Asthma Education and Prevention Program of the National Heart, Lung, and Blood Institute
P.O. Box 30105
Bethesda, MD 20824-0105
301-251-1222

National Cancer Institute
800-4-CANCER
A nationwide telephone service that provides information and referrals to local and regional resources. Callers are automatically connected to the nearest Cancer Information Service office.

National Center for Homeopathy
801 N. Fairfax Street, Suite 306
Alexandria, VA 22314
703-548-7790

National Certification Commission for Acupuncture and Oriental Medicine
1424 16th Street N.W., Suite 501
Washington, DC 20036
Phone: 202-232-1404
Web site: www.nccaom.org

National Chronic Fatigue Syndrome and Fibromyalgia Association
3521 Broadway, Suite 222
Kansas City, MO 64111
816-931-4777

National Clearinghouse for Alcohol and Drug Information
Box 2345
Rockville, MD 20847-2345
800-729-6686

National Commission for the Certification of Acupuncturists
919-787-5181

National Consumers League
815 15th Street N.W., Suite 516
Washington, DC 20005
202-639-8140

National Council of Senior Citizens
925 15th St. N.W.
Washington, DC 20005
202-347-8800

National Council on the Aging, Inc.
Dept. 5087
Washington, DC 20061-5087
800-867-2755

National Foundation for Depressive Illness
800-239-1263

National Headache Foundation
800-843 2256

National Heart, Lung, and Blood Institute Information Center
P.O. Box 30105
Bethesda, MD 20824-0105
301-251-1222

National Institute of Arthritis and Musculoskeletal and Skin Diseases
Information Clearinghouse
1 AMS Circle
Bethesda, MD 20892-3675
301-495-4484

National Institute of Medical Herbalists
56 Longbrook Street
Exeter, Devon EX4 6AH
England
Phone: 01392-426022
Fax: 01392-498963

National Institute of Mental Health
5600 Fishers Lane
Room 7C02
Rockville, MD 20857
301-443-4513
301-443-8431 (TDD)

National Institute of Neurological Disorders and Stroke
National Institutes of Health
31 Center Drive, MSC 2540
Building 31, Room 8A06
Bethesda, MD 20892-2540
800-352-9424

National Institute on Aging Information Center
P.O. Box 8057
Gaithersburg, MD 20898-8057
800-222-2225

National Jewish Center for Immunology and Respiratory Medicine
1400 Jackson Street
Denver, CO 80206
800-222-5864

National Medical Association (NMA)
1012 10th Street N.W.
Washington, DC 20001
202-347-1895

National Mental Health Association
800-969-NMHA

National Osteopathic Foundation
5775G Peachtree-Dunwoody Road, Suite 500
Atlanta, GA 30342

National Osteoporosis Foundation
1150 17th St. N.W., Suite 500
Washington, DC 20036
202-223-2226

National Rehabilitation Information Center
8455 Colesville Rd., #935
Silver Spring, MD 20910-3319
Toll free: 800-346-2742
Phone: 301-588-9284
Fax: 301-587-1967

National Self-Help Clearing House—CUNY
Graduate Center
33 W. 42nd St.
Room 1222
New York, NY 10036

National Senior Sports Association
10560 Main Street
Fairfax, VA 22030
703-758-8297

National Sleep Foundation
729 15th Street N.W., 4th Floor
Washington, DC 20005
202-347-3471

National Stroke Association
8480 E. Orchard Rd., Suite 1000
Englewood, CO 80110
800-787-6537

Naturopathic Medicine
The American Association of Naturopathic Physicians (AANP)
601 Valley Street, Suite 105
Seattle, WA 98109
206-298-0125

New England Herbal Supply Co.
299 Jagger Lane
Hebron, CT 06248
Toll free: 800-742-0631
Phone: 860-228-9705
Fax: 860-228-9705

North American Herbal Company
Nature's Solutions
P.O. Box 2945
Plattsburg, NY 12901-0269
800-644-5587

North American Spine Society
6300 N. River Rd., #115
Rosemont, IL 60018-4231
Phone: 708-698-1630
Fax: 708-823-8668

North American Vegetarian Society
P.O. Box 72
Dolgeville, NY 13329
518-568-7970

Office of Alternative Medicine Clearinghouse
P.O. Box 8218
Silver Spring, MD 20907-8218
Toll free: 888-644-6226
TTY/TDY: 888-644-6226
Fax: 301-495-4957
Web site: altmed.od.nih.gov

Oxford Health Plans
Personal Freedom Plan
Toll free: 800-444-6222

Reach to Recovery
c/o American Cancer Society
1599 Clifton Road, N.E.
Atlanta, GA 30329
800-422-6237

Respiratory Nursing Society (RNS)
5700 Old Orchard Road, First Floor
Skokie, IL 60077-1057
708-966-8673

Revitalizing Our Herbal Traditions
Box 746555
Arvada, CO 80006
Phone: 303-423-8800
Fax: 303-402-1564
E-mail: ahgoffice@earthlink.net

St. Anthony's Alternative Medicine Integration & Coverage
11410 Isaac Newton Square
Reston, VA 20190

Simon Foundation for Continence
Box 815
Wilmette, IL 60091
800-23-SIMON

The Society of Clinical and Experimental Hypnosis
3905 Vincennes Road, Suite 304
Indianapolis, IN 46268

Society of Clinical Hypnosis
2200 East Devon Avenue, Suite 291
Des Plaines, IL 60018

USDA Foreign Agricultural Service
Information Division, Room 5074-S
Washington, DC 20250-1000
Phone: 202-720-7115
Fax: 202-720-3229

USDA National Agricultural Library (NAL)
10301 Baltimore Blvd., Room 304
Beltsville, MD 20705-2351
301-504-6559

Vegetarian Resource Group
P.O. Box 1463
Baltimore, MD 21203
410-366-VEGE

Vermont Rehabilitation Engineering Research
Center for Low Back Pain
1 South Prospect Street
Burlington, VT 05401
Toll free: 800-527-7320
Phone: 802-656-4582 (voice/TDD)
Fax: 802-660-9243

Vinayak Ayurveda Center
2509 Virginia N.E., Suite D
Albuquerque, NM 87110
Phone: 505-296-6522
Fax: 505-298-2932

Weight-Control Information Network
1 Win Way
Bethesda, MD 20892-3665
Toll free: 800-946-8098
Phone: 301-570-2177
Fax: 301-570-2186

Appendix E

Glossary

ACTH (Adrenocorticotropic hormone) A hormone produced by the pituitary gland that stimulates adrenal glands to secrete the hormones they produce, including cortisone and cortisol.

Adrenal Pertaining to one or both glands located next to the kidneys. These glands secrete many hormones, including adrenaline, and play an important part in the body's endocrine system.

Adrenal glands Two glands attached to the kidneys. Each has an outer layer (cortex) that produces steroid hormones and an inner layer (medulla) that produces adrenaline.

Adrenaline A hormone produced by the adrenal glands that increases heart rate and prepares the body for crisis. Also called epinephrine.

Androgen One of a group of hormones, secreted by the testes and adrenal glands, that controls masculine sex characteristics, such as a deep voice, facial hair, and muscle bulk. Testosterone is the most important androgen. Women's adrenal glands and ovaries also secrete small amounts of androgens, but they do not have a strong masculinizing effect.

Andropause See Male menopause.

Angina pectoris See Angina.

Bladder The hollow organ that stores urine.

Burdock root A detoxifying herb that promotes healthy kidney function and helps to prevent water retention; helps to heal arthritis and rheumatism, and used as a blood purifier and cleanser.

Congenital venous leak A problem in men that occurs when the venous drainage system in the penis does not shut down properly during sexual arousal, resulting in the inability to maintain an erection. This problem can be corrected surgically, though usually without surgery.

Corpus cavernosa Part of the penis responsible for causing an erection; sometimes called "erection chambers."

Corpus spongiosum Penis Part of the penis that contains the urethra, through which urine passes from the bladder.

DHEA Anti-aging hormone sometimes called the mother hormone because the body converts it into estrogen and testosterone. DHEA raises sex hormones and is said to make you "feel younger and sexy."

Diurnal cycle In healthy people, hormone levels normally rise and fall in the bloodstream over a 24-hour period, following a natural, daily pattern called a diurnal cycle.

Ejaculate To eject sperm and seminal fluid.

Erectile dysfunction The frequent inability to achieve and maintain an erection suitable for sexual intercourse (see Impotence).

Erection The condition of erectile tissue when filled with blood, which then becomes hard and unyielding; denoting especially this state of the penis.

Genital herpes Viral infection of the genitals transmitted by intercourse or oral sex. Genital herpes may increase the risk of cervical cancer. Symptoms include painful blisters on the genitals that can cause painful urination, fever, malaise, and enlarged lymph glands. Currently incurable, but treatment can relieve symptoms.

Genitourinary tract The particular body system that forms, stores, and eliminates urine. Also has a role in male and female reproductive functions. Organs include the kidneys, ureters, bladder, urethra, uterus, fallopian tubes, ovaries, vagina, cervix, penis, scrotum, and testicles.

Gerson therapy A type of alternative medicine treatment that utilizes diet, detoxification, and therapeutic supplementation to reactivate and strengthen the immune system and restore the body's essential defenses.

Ginkgo biloba An herb that relaxes and opens up blood vessels, may increase male sexual performance and counteract male impotence, and also protects cell membranes from free radical damage, improving concentration and memory.

Ginseng An herb that is used to increase energy and relieve stress. May stimulate special enzymes that promote elimination of toxic foreign substances, as well as increase the immune response by stimulating the number of antibodies in the body.

Gland A group of special cells that make substances so that other parts of the body can work.

Glans penis The end portion of the penis, made up of the expansion of the corpus spongiosum penis.

Gonadal A term that pertains to gonads.

Gonadal impairment The decreased function of the gonads (testes in men, ovaries in women).

Gonadotropin Any hormone having a stimulating effect on the gonads.

Gonads Parts of the reproductive system that produce and release eggs (ovaries in the female) or sperm (testes in the male).

Gonorrhea Infectious disease of the reproductive organs and other body structures that is sexually transmitted (venereal disease). The most prominent symptom is a thick, green-yellow discharge from the penis or vagina. Antibiotics usually effect a cure.

Herpes Herpes type-1 causes common cold sores, which appear around the mouth. Herpes type-2 (HSV-2) is a viral infection of the genitals transmitted by sexual intercourse. Type-2 herpes infection can be transmitted to a newborn from an actively infected mother.

Hormones Powerful substances manufactured by the endocrine glands and carried by the blood to body tissues and organs. Hormones determine growth and structure of many organs (such as during growth and maturation) and also control many vital body functions. Too much or too little of a particular hormone can disrupt the process it controls.

Hypogonadism The subnormal activity of the gonads (testes in men, ovaries in women), the organs that produce sex hormones. In males, hypogonadism results in the decreased production of testosterone. The cause may lie in problems with the testes themselves or with the hypothalamus or pituitary, which produce hormones that stimulate the testes to produce testosterone.

Hypothalamus A part of the brain that controls various bodily functions, including hunger and thirst, body temperature, and some metabolic processes. In regulating male sexual functioning, the hypothalamus produces a hormone (gonadotrophin-releasing hormone, or GnRH) that stimulates the pituitary to produce another hormone (luteinizing hormone, or LH), which, in turn, signals the testes to produce testosterone. When the amount of testosterone in the bloodstream reaches a certain concentration, the hypothalamus decreases its production of GnRH.

Impotence The frequent inability to achieve and maintain an erection suitable for sexual intercourse (see Erectile dysfunction).

Intercourse Sexual relations or sexual coupling; coitus.

Klinefelter's syndrome An abnormality affecting the sexual development of boys. Males with this disorder have an extra chromosome that causes the process of puberty to be altered. Breasts enlarge and testes remain small, due to a near absence of testosterone. This disorder causes sterility because no sperm is produced. Testosterone replacement therapy can alleviate many of the symptoms of Klinefelter's syndrome.

Leydig cells Specific structures in the testes whose main function is to make testosterone. Before birth, Leydig cells supply testosterone to the developing fetus, which causes male genitals to develop. In men, these cells secrete testosterone in varying amounts until the end of life.

Libidinal A term relating to the libido.

Libido The emotional or psychic energy that in psychoanalytic theory is derived from primitive biological urges and that is usually goal-directed, sexual drive.

L-Lysine An amino acid that is also a cold sore preventer and may be effective against herpes.

Male menopause Symptoms, such as depression, change in libido, and impotence, in men at midlife. Many authorities claim no such condition exists.

Orchiectomy The surgical removal of the testicles, the major source of male hormones.

Orgasm The culmination of the sexual act.

Pituitary A gland located at the base of the brain that secretes several hormones that regulate growth and metabolism. These include two hormones: follicle-stimulating hormone (FSH) and luteinizing hormone (LH). When these hormones reach the testes, LH stimulates the production of testosterone and FSH stimulates the production of sperm.

Placebo effect A reaction that refers to the mysterious and uncharted mechanisms by which the power of suggestion can result in a physiological change, usually refers to case studies where participants are given "sugar pills" rather than the actual studied product.

Premature ejaculation The most common type of ejaculation problem, which usually means there is a shorter time before actual ejaculation than is normal or desired.

Quercetin A nutrient found in citrus fruits, red and yellow onions, and broccoli. Quercetin reduces inflammation associated with allergies, can inhibit the growth of head and neck cancers, and may reverse transcriptase, the method HIV uses to replicate itself.

Scrotum The pouch that encloses the testes in most male mammals.

Semen The penile ejaculate; a thick, yellowish-white, viscid fluid containing spermatozoa.

Seminal vesicles The pouches inside the body above the prostate that store semen.

Sexual intercourse Genital contact, the insertion of the penis into the vagina followed by ejaculation; coitus; copulation.

Sexuality The sum of a person's sexual behaviors and tendencies, and the strength of such tendencies.

Sexually Transmitted Disease (STD) Any disease acquired through sexual contact. There are currently more than 20 STDs identified, with millions of people being infected every year.

Sperm A male reproductive cell.

Spermatic fluid The male generative fluid; semen.

Sterility A term meaning the incapability of fertilization or reproduction.

Syphilis A contagious, sexually transmitted disease that causes widespread tissue destruction if not treated promptly. Syphilis is called "the great mimic" because its symptoms resemble those of many other diseases.

Testes The pair of male reproductive glands in the scrotum that are the source of sperm and the hormone testosterone. Also known as testicles or gonads.

Testicles In the male, two egg-shaped glands that produce sperm and sex hormones.

Testosterone The predominant male hormone. In addition to being essential to fertility, testosterone stimulates bone and muscle growth. It is also necessary for the development of male traits, such as a deep voice and facial hair. Female ovaries also produce minute amounts of testosterone before menopause.

Testosterone deficiency A condition that occurs when less than normal amounts of testosterone are secreted in males.

Urethra The tube running through the penis to the outside of the body. It carries urine from the bladder and semen from the sex glands.

Urethritis An inflammation or infection of the urethra.

Urinalysis A laboratory test performed on a urine sample that helps diagnose diseases of the kidney and other parts of the body.

Urinary bladder A muscular sac in the lower abdomen that stores urine brought to it from the kidneys by the ureters. The bladder stores urine until it can be eliminated through the urethra by contractions of the bladder muscles.

Urinary studies The laboratory or X-ray tests of the urinary tract.

Urinary tract The organs that produce, store, and eliminate urine. The organs are the kidneys, ureters, urinary bladder, and urethra.

Urogenital A term referring to the kidney and reproductive systems of the human body. Also called genitourinary.

Urologist A doctor who sees men and women for treatment of the urinary tract and men for treatment of the genital organs.

Venereal Related to sexual intercourse or sexual contact. Venereal diseases such as genital herpes, gonorrhea, or syphilis are now usually referred to as sexually transmitted diseases.

Virilization The process of developing masculine sexual characteristics. This occurs normally in boys. It may occur abnormally in women exposed to male sex hormones. Signs of virilization in women may include excessive hair growth, diminished or stopped menstruation, development of shoulder and arm muscles, and deepening of the voice.

Viropause See Male menopause.

Yohimbine An alkaloid, the bark of *Corynanthe yohimbi; it* has also been used for its alleged aphrodisiac properties.

Zoster Term used to describe a form of viral infection (herpes zoster, shingles) that often produces bands of painful blisters.

Index

A

D

E

F

G

I

K

L

O

P

Q

R

S

The *Unofficial Guide*™ Reader Questionnaire

If you would like to express your opinion about impotence or this guide, please complete this questionnaire and mail it to:

The *Unofficial Guide*™ Reader Questionnaire
Macmillan Lifestyle Group
1633 Broadway, Floor 7
New York, NY 10019-6785

Gender: ___ M ___ F

Age: ___ Under 30 ___ 31–40 ___ 41–50
___ Over 50

Education: ___ High school ___ College
___ Graduate/Professional

What is your occupation?

____

How did you hear about this guide?
___ Friend or relative
___ Newspaper, magazine, or Internet
___ Radio or TV
___ Recommended at bookstore
___ Recommended by librarian
___ Picked it up on my own
___ Familiar with the *Unofficial Guide*™ travel series

Did you go to the bookstore specifically for a book on impotence? Yes ___ No ___

Have you used any other *Unofficial Guides*™?
Yes ___ No ___

If Yes, which ones?

____
____
____

What other book(s) on impotence have you purchased?

____
____
____

Was this book:
___ more helpful than other(s)
___ less helpful than other(s)

Do you think this book was worth its price?
Yes ___ No ___

Did this book cover all topics related to impotence adequately? Yes ___ No ___

Please explain your answer:

____
____
____

Were there any specific sections in this book that were of particular help to you? Yes ___ No ___

Please explain your answer:

____
____
____

On a scale of 1 to 10, with 10 being the best rating, how would you rate this guide? ___

What other titles would you like to see published in the *Unofficial Guide*™ series?

____
____

Are *Unofficial Guides*™ readily available in your area? Yes ___ No ___

Other comments:

____
____
____
____

Get the inside scoop...with the Unofficial Guides™!

The Unofficial Guide to Alternative Medicine
ISBN: 0-02-862526-9 Price: $15.95

The Unofficial Guide to Buying a Home
ISBN: 0-02-862461-0 Price: $15.95

The Unofficial Guide to Buying or Leasing a Car
ISBN: 0-02-862524-2 Price: $15.95

The Unofficial Guide to Childcare
ISBN: 0-02-862457-2 Price: $15.95

The Unofficial Guide to Cosmetic Surgery
ISBN: 0-02-862522-6 Price: $15.95

The Unofficial Guide to Dieting Safely
ISBN: 0-02-862521-8 Price: $15.95

The Unofficial Guide to Eldercare
ISBN: 0-02-862456-4 Price: $15.95

The Unofficial Guide to Hiring Contractors
ISBN: 0-02-862460-2 Price: $15.95

The Unofficial Guide to Investing
ISBN: 0-02-862458-0 Price: $15.95

The Unofficial Guide to Planning Your Wedding
ISBN: 0-02-862459-9 Price: $15.95

All books in the *Unofficial Guide*™ series are available at your local bookseller, or by calling 1-800-428-5331.

About the Authors

Debra Fulghum Bruce and Dr. Harris H. McIlwain can tell you everything you need to know about impotence. Debra is a Florida-based health journalist pursuing a Ph.D. in Health Communications. Debra has written over 2,500 articles for women's and health magazines, such as *Woman's Day, Prevention,* and *Success.* She is the author or co-author of 38 books, and her promotional ventures include ongoing weekly seminars and a new fitness video, *Flexible Fitness: An Arthritis Workout,* starring Linda Lavin.

Dr. Harris H. McIlwain was rated one of the top 100 physicians in America by *Town and Country* magazine in 1997. He currently works at the Tampa Medical Group in Tampa, Florida. He has held appointments at many Florida hospitals, including St. Joseph's Hospital, University Community Hospital, Tampa General Hospital, Humana Hospital Brandon, and Town and Country Hospital. Dr. McIlwain is certified by the American Board of Internal Medicine in Rheumatology and Internal Medicine.

Together, Debra and Dr. McIlwain have written 13 other health books, including *The Unofficial Guide to Alternative Medicine, Super Calcium Counter, The Osteoporosis Cure, The Fibromyalia Handbook, Winning with Arthritis, Winning with Back Pain,* and *Stop Osteoarthritis Now.*